Effective Secondary Prevention and Cardiac Rehabilitation

Titles of related interest in the UK Key Advances in Clinical Practice Series

Clinical Governance and the NHS Reforms: Enabling Excellence or Imposing Control?

NICE, CHI and the NHS Reforms: Enabling Excellence or Imposing Control?

Effective Secondary Prevention and Cardiac Rehabilitation

Edited by

David Wood MSc FRCP FRCPE FFPHM FESC
Professor of Cardiovascular Medicine, National Heart and Lung Institute, Imperial College School of Medicine, London, UK

Andrew McLeod MA MB BChir MD FRCP FESC
Immediate Past President of the British Association for Cardiac Rehabilitation and Consultant Cardiologist, Poole Hospital, Dorset, UK

Mark Davis MB ChB MRCGP DRCOG DOccMed
Founding Chairman, Primary Care Cardiovascular Society and Member, CHD Task Force, Department of Health, Leeds, UK

Andrew Miles MSc MPhil PhD
Professor of Public Health Policy and UK Key Advances Series Organiser, University of East London, UK

UeL University Centre for Public Health Policy & Health Services Research

British Cardiac Society

Primary Care Cardiovascular Society

Society of Cardiothoracic Surgeons

British Association of Cardiac Rehabilitation

AESCULAPIUS MEDICAL PRESS
LONDON SAN FRANCISCO SYDNEY

Published by

Aesculapius Medical Press (London, San Francisco, Sydney)
Centre for Public Health Policy and Health Services Research
School of Health Sciences
University of East London
33 Shore Road, London E9 7TA, UK

First published 2002

British Library Cataloguing in Publication Data
A catalogue record for this book is available from the British Library

ISBN 1 903044 22 7

While the advice and information in this book are believed to be true and accurate at the time of going to press, neither the authors nor the publishers nor the sponsoring institutions can accept any legal responsibility or liability for any errors or omissions that may be made. In particular (but without limiting the generality of the preceding disclaimer) every effort has been made to check drug usages; however, it is possible that errors have been missed. Furthermore, dosage schedules are constantly being revised and new side effects recognised. For these reasons, the reader is strongly urged to consult the drug companies' printed instructions before administering any of the drugs recommended in this book.

Further copies of this volume are available from:
Claudio Melchiorri
Research Dissemination Fellow
Centre for Public Health Policy and Health Services Research
School of Health Sciences
University of East London
33 Shore Road, London E9 7TA, UK

Fax: 020 8525 8661
email: claudio@keyadvances4.demon.co.uk

Typeset, printed and bound in Britain
Peter Powell Origination and Print Limited

Contents

Contributors

Hugh JN Bethell MD FRCP FRCGP, General Practitioner, Alton, Hampshire

D John Betteridge BSc PhD MD FRCP, Professor of Endocrinology and Metabolism, Department of Medicine, The Middlesex Hospital, London

John C Chambers MB BS MRCP, Lecturer in Cardiology, National Heart and Lung Institute at Charing Cross Campus, Imperial College School of Medicine, London

Carol Fisher MB BS MRCP, Clinical Research Fellow, Department of Cardiology, Western Infirmary, Glasgow

Jaspal S Kooner MD FRCP, Consultant Cardiologist, Hammersmith Hospital, London

Andrew A McLeod MA MB BChir MD FRCP FESC, Consultant Cardiologist, Poole Hospital, and President of the British Association for Cardiac Rehabilitation

John JV McMurray MD FRCP, Professor of Medical Cardiology, Department of Cardiology, Western Infirmary, Glasgow

Sheila Ryan RGN RHV, Cardiac Rehabilitation Co-ordinator, Newham Primary Care Trust, London

Adam D Timmis MD FRCP, Consultant Cardiologist, St Bartholomew's and the Royal London NHS Trust, The London Chest Hospital, London

Tom Treasure MS MD FRCS, Professor of Cardiothoracic Surgery, GKT Medical School at Guy's Hospital, London

Hugh Tunstall-Pedoe MD FFPHM FRCP, Professor of Cardiovascular Epidemiology, Ninewells Hospital, University of Dundee at Ninewells Hospital, Scotland

David Wood, MSc FRCP FRCPE FFPHM FESC, Garfield Weston Chair of Cardiovascular Medicine, National Heart and Lung Institute at Charing Cross Campus, Imperial College School of Medicine, London

Preface

Prevention means 'to act in anticipation of a future event . . . to preclude, stop or hinder'. It is therefore not a metaphysical absolute, but rather a term that can be applied to anything that diminishes, delays or abolishes risk or individual probability of onset of disease, progression of disease or consequence of disease such as death and disability. Prevention is therefore risk reduction. Narrowing of the coronary arteries progresses for decades before precipitating myocardial infarction (MI) when clinical disease will become manifest, often with catastrophic consequences. However, half of all major coronary events occur in those with previously diagnosed coronary heart disease, a high-risk subset of the population. In these individuals, there is huge potential for risk reduction by influencing processes in both the myocardium and the coronary arteries. This, if achieved, is *effective secondary prevention.*

If this is how we might define effective secondary prevention, how might we define effective cardiac rehabilitation, a process that must be put in place after an event, which for whatever reason could not be precluded? Overviews of cardiac rehabilitation services published in 1988, for example, suggested that cardiac rehabilitation could reduce mortality after MI by 20–25%, conclusions based on data that had accumulated from much earlier years. The development of services drawing on these data have, incontrovertibly, led to very substantial improvements in both morbidity and mortality in patients with coronary artery disease through use of therapies such as β blockade, antiplatelet drugs, angiotensin-converting enzyme inhibitors and hydroxymethylglutaryl-coenzyme A (HMG-CoA) reductase inhibitors. Agreed, the relevance of rehabilitation efforts derived from studies in some cases dating back 30 years or more must be revisited and questioned, but there are many opportunities for the development of comprehensive rehabilitation programmes that will address risk factors holistically, and these need to be urgently addressed. Indeed, the British Heart Foundation estimates that, in comparison with the 150,000 or so survivors of MI per year in the UK, there are three times as many patients with heart failure and an order of magnitude greater number of patients with angina pectoris, the majority managed within the primary care setting. Strategies that seek comprehensively to implement established treatment regimens and to provide access to such services to all who are judged to need then will lead to the development of *effective cardiac rehabilitation.* Parts 1–4 of this volume review current epidemiological data, together with a thorough documentation and discussion of the current scientific evidence and expert opinion base underpinning the place of non-pharmacological intervention, medical and surgical interventions.

Effective secondary prevention for patients with acute coronary syndromes requires an appropriate infrastructure for its delivery, involving dedicated cardiologists and cardiac nurses to review patients in the coronary care unit setting, prescribe drugs of proven value for secondary prevention and deliver lifestyle advice. Staff and facilities are also required for outpatient review, rehabilitation courses, home visits and smoking cessation clinics. Finally, patient self-help groups need to be established in order that early momentum is maintained in the longer term. It must be remembered that, traditionally, such programmes have been offered to patients after an MI, or after cardiac surgery, and not to those with other clinical manifestations of coronary artery disease, thus excluding about half of all patients with symptomatic coronary disease in the community. Patients with exertional angina are at high risk of progressing to unstable angina or MI, or of dying from this disease, and should therefore be eligible for a comprehensive cardiac prevention and rehabilitation programme. Parts 5 and 6 examine these issues in considerable detail.

It is well established that risk differs as a function of ethnicity, and effective services will need to take this strongly into account. Coronary heart disease (CHD) in UK south-east Asian subgroups is 40% higher compared with that in Europeans, although the high mortality is not uniform among Indians, Pakistanis and Bangladeshis. Previous studies have suggested that the prevalence of diabetes is higher, and that of smoking, hypercholesterolaemia and hypertension lower, in south-east Asian subgroups than in Europeans, implying that classic risk factors do not account for the higher CHD mortality among Asians. However, there are important differences in the prevalence of coronary risk factors among south-east Asian subgroups, and compared with those in Europeans. Strategies for reducing risk among south-east Asian subgroups include identification of patients with established vascular disease, their first-degree relatives, and those with diabetes, central obesity and an additional risk factor. Ensuring the identification of at-risk individuals and guaranteeing access and equity to effective prevention and rehabilitation services to the population at large form the focus of Part 6.

In the current age, where doctors and health professionals are increasingly overwhelmed by clinical information, we have aimed to provide a fully current, fully referenced text which is as succinct as possible but as comprehensive as necessary, placing detailed reviews of scientific evidence and expert opinion for effective cardiac prevention and rehabilitation within the context of service delivery as a whole and with reference to the modern policy requirements of the NHS, specifically with regard to the National Service Framework for Coronary Heart Disease. Consultants in cardiology and general medicine and their trainees, and general practitioners and their trainees, are likely to find it of particular value as part of their continuing professional development and specialist training, respectively, and we advance it explicitly as an excellent tool for these purposes. We anticipate, however, that the book will prove of substantial use to cardiac nurse specialists and to all those other pivotal members of the multidisciplinary clinical team with a responsibility for or interest in the provision of effective, efficient services for cardiac prevention and rehabilitation.

In conclusion we thank Parke-Davis Medical Ltd for a grant of educational sponsorship which helped organise a national symposium held with the British

Cardiac Society, the British Association for Cardiac Rehabilitation, the Society of Cardiothoracic Surgeons and the Primary Care Cardiovascular Society at the Royal College of Physicians of London, at which synopses of the constituent chapters of the current volume were delivered.

David Wood MSc FRCP FRCPE FFPHM FESC
Andrew McLeod MA MB BChir MD FRCP FESC
Mark Davis MB ChB MRCGP DRCOG DOccMed
Andrew Miles MSc MPhil PhD

PART 1

Prevention of coronary heart disease

Chapter 1

What was preventing coronary heart disease prevention and why its time has now come

Hugh Tunstall-Pedoe

Introduction

Publication of *The National Service Framework for Coronary Heart Disease* (Department of Health 2000) in England marks national recognition of the need for systematic implementation of both primary and secondary prevention of coronary heart disease (CHD). The author's aim here is to explain earlier confusion and scepticism over causation and prevention, why they prevented action and why they still matter. Without discussing directly the randomised controlled trials (RCTs) on which evidence is now based, the author describes some important results from recent major epidemiological studies. These corroborate the promised impact of the interventions that are now becoming generalised.

Sceptical arguments about prevention are still important because they were widely repeated in public until very recently. They still lurk close to the surface, like fossils, in the confused thinking of many people. These include those whose fervour for prevention is at best lukewarm, in the medical professions, readers of broadsheet newspapers, and among medical and lay journalists, but also those who appear enthusiastic but have never thought through their sometimes contradictory ideas. The author has called these arguments 'dinosaurs' teeth'.

Dinosaurs' teeth and the prevention of prevention

There are four fossil dinosaurs' teeth that warrant discussion:

1. Prevention is not orthodox medicine.
2. Prevention is all or nothing. Delaying or slowing the onset or progression of a disease is not prevention.
3. You should not interfere with disease mechanisms or risk factors if you do not fully understand them.
4. Unknown risk factors are more important than the known ones.

These views are still believed by many but were very publicly promoted 15 years ago. As the author stated while participating in a sponsored medical debate in the Oxford Union at that time on the proposal 'Risk factors are best left alone', these attitudes were very British and combined intellectual arrogance with complete impotence. They were promoted by leading academics, pleading that we needed not action but more research. British medicine and cardiology were conservative and backward in their lack of enthusiasm for public action to prevent coronary disease. To its credit, however, British medicine was responsible for pioneering the RCT in the late 1940s. British cardiology in the early 1980s led the initiation and collaboration in very large trials that provided the evidence for secondary prevention. British medicine and cardiology were therefore major contributors to the establishment of evidence-based medicine. Many of the dinosaur ideas, greatly respected in their day, now appear antediluvian precisely because they were drowned in the flood of ISIS and other large studies published during the miraculous decade from the early 1980s to the mid-1990s.

Prevention is not orthodox medicine

When the author began research in cardiovascular epidemiology in 1970 there was little conclusive evidence, other than for cardiopulmonary resuscitation, that preventive or therapeutic measures could substantially prevent CHD or change its natural history once it was established. Treatment was of symptoms. This applied equally well to almost all of the other so-called chronic diseases. Physicians historically had always existed to diagnose and treat patients and, for centuries, had been specifically prevented by professional rules from advertising themselves or their treatments. On the other hand, unlicensed quacks (short for quack-salvers), mountebanks and charlatans were free to peddle their unproven and expensive nostrums publicly, such as elixirs of life and snake oil. They made extravagant claims for cure or prevention – a phenomenon still seen in much of the coverage of so-called 'health correspondents' in the Sunday newspaper supplements, and on the internet. Much of what would now be labelled 'health promotion' had always been unsubstantiated pseudo-science, and fraudulent commercial self-promotion. This explains the traditional scepticism and antagonism of the physician to dramatic public claims of prevention, even though, inevitably, this sometimes applied to advice that turned out subsequently to be correct.

Scepticism about prevention became unjustified for infectious diseases before this happened in the chronic 'degenerative' diseases. Edward Jenner of the eighteenth century is not now honoured because he repeated old wives' tales about the immunity to smallpox of milkmaids who had suffered from cowpox. Others had done so before him. What made him exceptional was that he carried out rigorous experiments on humans to test the assertion, and thereby placed vaccination for smallpox in the domain of what is now called evidence-based medicine. This led to the idea of specific germs and specific immunity for infectious diseases and to routine immunisation against childhood and other illnesses. Within medicine a new discipline of public health became concerned with immunisation and prevention, with ramifications into general practice. Hospital doctors, the specialists, were still concerned with the diagnosis and treatment of chronic degenerative diseases that patently had not, and mostly could not, be prevented. They were also, inevitably, furthest removed from the social and environmental factors that generated these diseases. Lack of involvement with prevention was not necessarily true of all specialties, e.g. the antenatal clinic in obstetrics is concerned with little else but prevention. The modern diabetic clinic is intimately concerned with prevention of diabetic complications, through identification and control of risk factors.

Within the last generation, the face of medicine has been radically changed. It is now possible, to a large extent, to prevent the onset and the progression of some chronic diseases using interventions proven by RCTs. Traditional attitudes are undergoing a profound revolution. Indeed this is sometimes in danger of going too far. Planning and working to prevent disease is of fundamental importance. However, it would be naïve not to accept that, in most clinical situations, what the patient wants and expects is efficient diagnosis of what he or she already has, plus a full explanation, including the prognosis, followed by measures to relieve the symptoms, whether or not life is actually extended. Enthusiasm for changing the incidence and natural history of disease and improving its statistics should not be at the expense of traditional medical roles.

Prevention is all or nothing, so that delaying or slowing the onset or progression of a disease is not prevention

There is a widespread misconception that, if a disease is still occurring at all, or its onset is delayed, it is not being prevented. If that argument were valid then the only disease that might have been prevented would be smallpox. For proof we would have to wait until everybody who was alive, at the time that the World Health Organization announced the end of smallpox around 1980, had died without developing it. This is an extreme and impractical viewpoint.

Disease in the population is measured by epidemiological disease rates such as incidence and mortality. Each of these measures incorporates the idea of a numerator – cases related to a conventional denominator – the at-risk population and a time period – most usually one year. These disease rates are measures of population risk, or individual probability if applied to an individual. In these terms there is nothing mystical or metaphysical about prevention. *Prevention is reduction in risk – anything and everything that reduces risk is prevention.* The risk being considered may be the first development of the clinical disease (reduced by primary prevention) or progression of the disease after it is recognised (reduced by secondary prevention).

In the case of coronary heart disease we can represent this conceptually as two separate progressions: one in the wall of the coronary artery and the second in the muscle of the heart, the myocardium. In the first, atheromatous plaques are developing in the wall of the coronary arteries over several decades in an individual who has no symptoms because nothing is happening in the myocardium. When myocardial ischaemia (angina pectoris) or myocardial infarction occurs (the second progression), the patient now has coronary heart disease and the era of primary prevention ends. Secondary prevention is likewise concerned with attempting to slow the progression of atheromatous disease in the coronary arteries. in addition, however, it attempts to modify or ameliorate further damage to the myocardium. Primary and secondary prevention are in a continuum as far as the coronary arteries are concerned – the coronary artery is, if you like, unaware of what is happening in the myocardium. However, the latter, and the increased risk, provide additional opportunities and modalities for risk reduction, inapplicable in primary prevention where only the coronary artery is involved and the risk is much smaller.

Primary prevention will ideally target the whole population whereas secondary prevention involves only those with known vascular disease, so its remit is far less ambitious but much more focused. However, a disputed proportion (somewhere between 10 and 30 per cent) of those experiencing their first manifestation of coronary disease will die suddenly as they do so. These unfortunates will be beyond the scope of secondary prevention.

Reduction of risk may result in either an event not happening at all or delay in its occurrence. Either of these is prevention. The epidemic of coronary heart disease after the Second World War saw a massive increase in premature CHD occurring in young people. It is now being pushed back into old age where it previously belonged. A comparison of CHD mortality in men and women tells a similar story. Mortality is some four times higher in men than in women in early middle age, the ratio falling to approximately 1.6 in old age (Tunstall-Pedoe 1998). Partly because of this, women live longer than men so that they account for the majority of coronary deaths over the age of 75. Their lifetime cumulative coronary risk is not too different from that in men, but it is nonsense to suggest that therefore there is no difference in actual risk between them. If coronary disease could be prevented in men so that their incidence and mortality risks were the same as those in women, this would be a monumental achievement, not to be minimised by equating risks over unequal time periods.

One specific example of a delayed effect that may account for some of the confusion is where a palliative procedure results in an initial survival advantage, lost after some years by a 'catching up' effect in the treatment group. Although it is true that a temporary advantage is less satisfactory than one that is sustained, even a temporary advantage represents diminished medium-term risk, equivalent to prevention and enhanced survival. Ultimately everybody dies.

You should not interfere with disease mechanisms or risk factors if you do not fully understand them

This was the basis of an intellectually formidable Professor of Medicine's British Heart Foundation-funded touring lecture in the 1980s. 'Should every cow carry a government health warning?' The basis of this was 'leave cholesterol alone, you do not know what you are doing. There will be all sorts of unfortunate consequences.'

Although there is much to be said for prudence, there are no diseases in which we can claim that we fully understand all the mechanisms, because there are always wheels within wheels. Edward Jenner described the prevention of smallpox 150 years before viruses were identified and described. Although medical science improved the production and harvesting of vaccine and was able eventually to visualise viruses under the electron microscope, and demonstrate their nucleic acid content, it was Jenner's pragmatic technique, applied systematically, that eventually abolished the disease two centuries later.

Part of the Professor of Medicine's message was in fact pandering to the idea, taken from the germ theory of disease, that every disease had a fundamental cause, such as a virus, but it was mistaken in implying that without knowing the 'real cause' nothing effective can be done. The conclusion, repeatedly, was that what was needed was more research, rather than action. His final sop to prevention was, however, to state that we should concentrate on campaigning against smoking. The author pointed out, when he came to Dundee, pursuing his own argument, that we did not really know how or why cigarette smoking caused either coronary heart disease or bronchial carcinoma. Should we not wait until we had done a lot more research on the subject? Interfering with mechanisms that we did not understand, by stopping people smoking, might have unforeseen consequences! However, his scepticism did not extend to the campaign against cigarette smoking. This was a safe target for two decades before cholesterol became one – possibly because the majority of doctors did not then smoke.

Cholesterol was identified as a risk factor in American studies in the 1950s, but it was very reluctantly accepted on this side of the Atlantic. Cholesterol was looked on as an example of American paranoia and hypochondria. It was definitely not British to talk about cholesterol or admit that you had had it measured. Around 1972 the author was considered to be a freak by the BBC science correspondent interviewing him. 'Oh, you're a cholesterol man!' As late as 1993 a leading cardiologist could claim at a seminar on epidemiology and prevention organised by the British Cardiac Society that 'The BMJ has now proved that cardiologists can forget about cholesterol'. He was referring to a spate of negative articles suggesting that low cholesterol was associated with accidents, violence and suicide, following earlier ones questioning bowel and other cancer. The author's daughter was interviewed for entry to Oxford medical school at about that time. Questioned about coronary risk factors her mention of cholesterol met the response 'What about the Masai?'. Eskimos also figured in such debates and the author guesses the man in the moon would also have qualified. Such opinions were abruptly terminated by a series of RCT results of lipid lowering using statins, in both primary and secondary prevention. These showed that cholesterol lowering was associated with commensurate reductions in vascular disease and deaths from all causes without obvious associated dangers (see later chapters).

Scepticism and questioning of causation and prevention of coronary heart disease was academically much more respectable than championing it. Champions of prevention were accused of lack of judgement and emotional arguments. The pragmatic position the author adopted – that in a war where you are taking heavy casualties you do not sit on your hands but take reasonable measures to reduce risk, if you know that they are practical, feasible and likely to be safe – was obstructed by the influence of eminent dinosaurs. As another retired Professor of Medicine, charged with finding out about diet, put it to me in the middle 1980s: 'This is all very controversial. Don't you agree we would be much better doing nothing?'

Unknown risk factors are more important than the known ones

It is true that a good definition of a wise man is someone who knows the limitations of his own knowledge. However, this particular dinosaur tooth is again a policy of despair and a prescription for impotence. It panders to an extremely common misconception about how risk and risk factors operate. Many of those untrained in epidemiology visualise the effect of risk factors as additive. Figure 1.1 shows that, if you have five risk factors, each scored 2, and you reduce the value of one of the two known ones from 2 to 1, an additive model would reduce the total risk from 10 to 9 units. Similar reduction in a second factor would reduce risk to 8, only 20 per cent down from the original value. Contrast that with a multiplicative model of risk where each factor doubles the risk (Figure 1.2). The fifth power of 2 is 32. Halving the contribution of one risk factor would drop risk from 32 to 16 (50 per cent) and halving a second one would reduce it further to 8. This 75 per cent reduction in risk is occurring without any change in the majority, three out of five, of the risk factors. The multiplicative model of risk means that the total number of known and unknown risk factors is unimportant provided that effective measures of controlling one or two are available. Unlike the additive model, the risk is not specific to particular factors so that the same risk product can be diminished by several different means. The multiplicative model is at the heart of most risk factor formulae developed to explain risk, as they work on a logarithmic or quasi-logarithmic scale (Anderson *et al.* 1991; Tunstall-Pedoe 1991). Risk in the real world appears to follow a multiplicative pattern more than an additive one, although sometimes it seems to operate in between. (see tables in Kannel *et al.* 1986). What this all means is that you do not have to know everything about a disease in order to prevent it effectively – i.e. reduce its risk by 80 per cent or so. This is the same conclusion we reached after extracting the previous dinosaur tooth!

Potential size of the target for secondary prevention

The incidence (new disease rates) and prevalence (proportion of the population affected) increase with age. Both are sensitive to exactly how they are defined. If a cut-off of age 65 is used, we have found in the Scottish MONICA population of

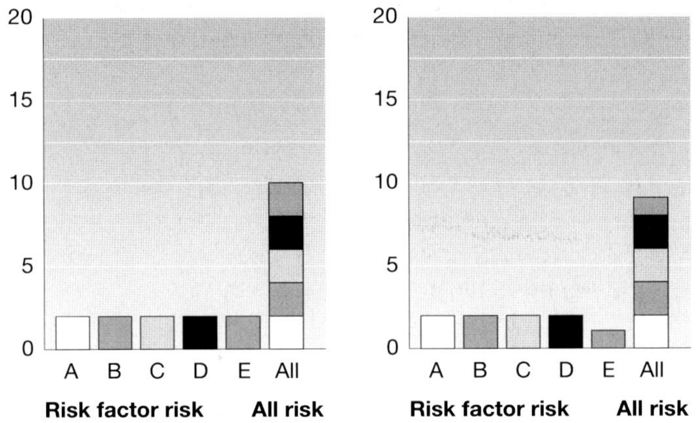

Figure 1.1 Additive model of action of coronary risk factors

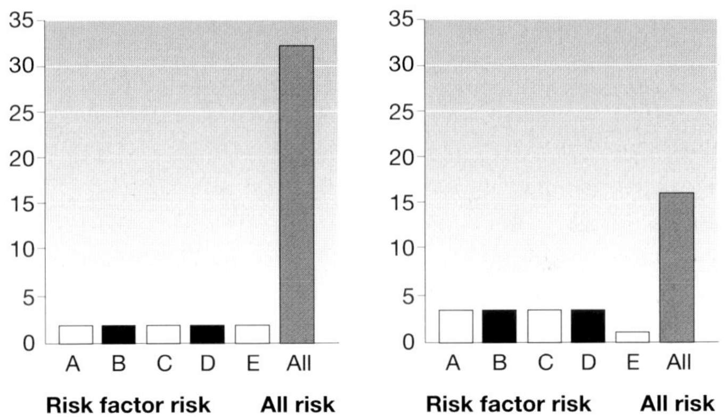

Figure 1.2 Multiplicative model of coronary risk factors

Glasgow (Tunstall-Pedoe *et al.* 1996b) that approximately half of all identified episodes of myocardial infarction or coronary death occur in men and women with a previous history of coronary heart disease – either angina pectoris or non-fatal infarction (Table 1.1). The other half are new events. This means that half of coronary events can only be prevented by primary prevention but it means also that half, in this age group, are candidates for secondary prevention. As the prevalence of previous coronary disease in the population is many times below half (see next paragraph) this means that those with previous CHD are many times more likely to suffer an event. They are at high risk, and should be identified and known to their usual medical attendants in order to have special measures taken. This is part of what the National Service Framework is about.

Table 1.1 Previous medical history in men and women with myocardial infarction or coronary deaths below age 65 (Glasgow MONICA Project 1985–1991)

	Men (%) *(n = 3,991)*	*Women (%)* *(n = 1,551)*
Myocardial infarction	32	25
Angina pectoris	42	40
Any CHD	49	46

The previous analysis was the retrospective history obtained at the time of a heart attack. It is possible to look at the same problem prospectively in the Scottish Heart Health study in which 10,000 men and women were screened for risk factors, including evidence of CHD, and then followed for future coronary events (Tunstall-Pedoe *et al.* 1997). Table 1.2 shows the hazard ratio for coronary deaths of subjects with no evidence of CHD at baseline (given a value of one) with those with varying evidence of CHD followed for an average of 7.6 years. Those with angina or infarction at baseline make up a small proportion of the population but account for a large proportion of the subsequent deaths and they are therefore at very high risk. Note, however, that Table 1.2 would include those who developed angina or infarction during the follow-up as being disease free at baseline, so the real contrast would be even greater.

Table 1.2 includes an interesting intermediate group of cases who might be the subject of screening and intervention at some time in the future. They do not have diagnosed angina or previously diagnosed myocardial infarction (the final two columns of the table) but do have positive responses to a Rose chest pain questionnaire, or that and ECG findings compatible with myocardial ischaemia. Their risk is greater than that in those without CHD but lower than that in those with diagnosed CHD. (The values in men are more stable and reliable because they are based on larger numbers of events than in women.) There is no obvious term for something between primary and secondary prevention. Intermediary means something else. Possible terms might be intermediate, post-primary or pre-secondary. My own preference

Table 1.2 Hazard ratio of coronary death by evidence of CHD at baseline (men and women aged 40–59 followed for 7.6 years in the Scottish Heart Health Study)

	None	*Rose angina*	*ECG positive*	*Angina history*	*Myocardial infarction history*
Men (%)	78.5	6.4	6.9	3.4	4.8
159 deaths (hazard ratio)	1	1.9	3.8	5.4	8.0
Women (%)	79.1	7.7	8.2	3.4	1.6
47 deaths (hazard ratio)	1	1.9	5.4	3.8	25.3

would be post-primary prevention. Although this is a high-risk group, neither the ECG findings nor the chest-pain questionnaire results are free from considerable dilution with false positives who do not have CHD. This explains why figures are so similar for men and women despite their differences in risk. These screening findings are potentially valuable markers for intensified prevention, but the danger of false labelling should be recognised because these findings are not diagnostic, alone, for CHD.

How the WHO MONICA project results corroborate secondary prevention

The WHO MONICA project was an observational study and not an RCT, so that its findings do not have the same degree of conviction for causality as do RCTs. What it does do, however, is to show what is happening in defined populations in association with different risk factors and drugs over time. There is always a worry as to how the results of RCTs extrapolate to the real world, as their subjects are often a subset of those to whom treatments are then extrapolated.

In the Glasgow population (Tunstall-Pedoe *et al.* 1996a) we have shown that men and women with a previous history of CHD have a higher in-hospital fatality rate from myocardial infarction than those without such a history, but this difference is compensated for to some extent in that the fitter men and women, without previous CHD, have relatively more of their deaths suddenly, before reaching hospital. The overall case fatality from onset to 28 days is fairly similar whether or not there is a previous history of CHD. Equally interesting is the comparison of men and women who have a previous history of CHD (nearly half the total, see Table 1.1) and either are, or are not, on therapy at the time of their new event. The treatment included aspirin, nitrates, β blockers and calcium blockers (there is so much overlap that our initial analyses could not readily disentangle separate effects). Analyses showed confusing results for the impact of prior treatment on hospital-related fatality rates. However, there is a clear and consistent picture in both sexes that the drugs used for secondary prevention were associated with fewer sudden deaths outside hospital and more survivors from coronary events overall. Figure 1.3 shows results in men. As a descriptive analysis, we could not, however, prove that the drugs were changing the risks of sudden death directly, as there might be other factors operating to distinguish the two groups. However, the results are highly suggestive and strongly reinforce the virtues of prophylactic secondary prevention, not in this case in preventing recurrence, but in reducing the sudden death component and the 28-day fatality of such recurrences.

Comparison across the MONICA populations is even more suggestive of the benefits of drug use in coronary care, whether acutely or in secondary prevention. Those populations that had the largest increase in usage of coronary drugs (such as aspirin, β blockers, angiotensin-converting enzyme or ACE inhibitors, thrombolytic

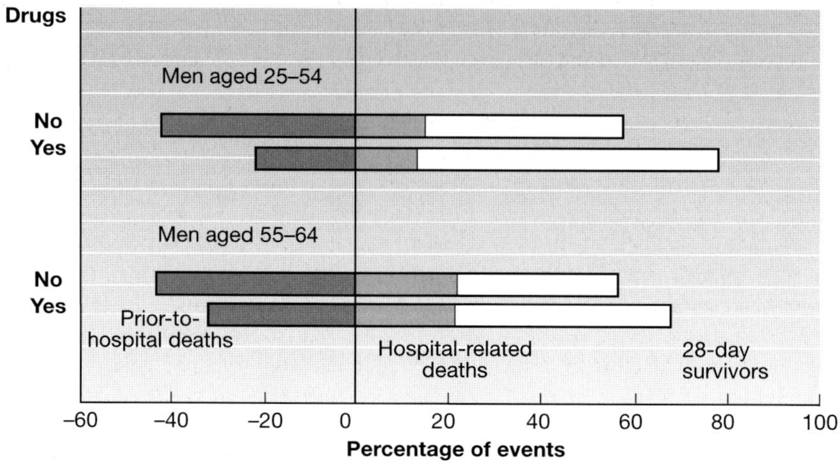

Figure 1.3 Pattern of pre- and hospital-related mortality in coronary events in relation to cardiovascular medication before onset. (Note each bar totals 100%.) Cases are those with previous history of CHD (Glasgow MONICA Project)

therapy and also coronary revascularisation) also had the largest reductions in CHD mortality during the decade of the mid-1980s to the mid-1990s. Again the results are not proof. They are so powerful that they are almost too good to be true. But they are a very strong positive corroboration of the potential benefits of the obsessional application of secondary preventive measures (Tunstall-Pedoe *et al.* 2000).

Conclusion

This chapter has described the theoretical background to both primary and secondary prevention. It has exposed some of the conceptual errors that have prevented positive thinking on the subject. It has also shown the potential scope for secondary prevention. Without entering into results of randomised controlled trials, it has shown that both local (Glasgow) and collaborative results from the WHO MONICA project, the largest observational study of CHD ever undertaken, are fully supportive of the importance and potential for secondary prevention.

References

Anderson KM, Wilson PWF, Odell PM, Kannel WB (1991). An updated coronary risk profile: a statement for health professionals. *Circulation* **83**, 356–362

Department of Health (2000). *National Service Framework for Coronary Heart Disease.* London: Department of Health

Kannel WB, Neaton JD, Wentworth D *et al.* (1986) Overall and coronary heart disease mortality rates in relation to major risk factors in 352,348 men screened for MRFIT. *American Heart Journal* **112**, 825–836

Tunstall-Pedoe H (1991). The Dundee coronary risk-disk for management of change in risk factors. *British Medical Journal* **303**, 744–747

Tunstall-Pedoe H (1998). Myth and paradox of coronary risk and the menopause. *The Lancet* **351**, 1425–1427

Tunstall-Pedoe H, Morrison C, Woodward M (1996a). 28-day case fatality of coronary events and the proportion of out of hospital deaths in relation to age, sex and previous coronary heart disease (CHD): the Glasgow MONICA Project. *British Heart Journal* **75**, 203

Tunstall-Pedoe H, Morrison C, Woodward M, Fitzpatrick B, Watt G (1996b). Sex differences in myocardial infarction and coronary deaths in the Scottish MONICA population of Glasgow 1985–91: presentation, diagnosis, treatment, and 28-day case fatality of 3991 events in men and 1551 events in women. *Circulation* **93**, 1981–1992

Tunstall-Pedoe H, Woodward M, Tavendale R, A'Brook R, McCluskey MK (1997). Comparison of the prediction by 27 different factors of coronary heart disease and death in men and women of the Scottish heart health study: cohort study. *British Medical Journal* **315**, 722–729

Tunstall-Pedoe H, Vanuzzo D, Hobbs M *et al.* for WHO Monica Project (2000). Estimation of the contribution of changes in coronary care to improving survival, event rates, and coronary heart disease mortality across the WHO MONICA Project. *The Lancet* **355**, 688–700

PART 2

Evidence and opinion for non-pharmacological intervention

Chapter 2

Evidentiary basis for non-pharmacological intervention – effective management of lifestyle and associated risk factors

Andrew A McLeod

If you have built castles in the air, your work need not be lost; that is where they should be. Now put foundations under them.

Henry David Thoreau

Introduction

Patients with cardiovascular disease, particularly ischaemic heart disease, can expect reduced risk of complications after their first cardiac event by virtue of an impressive array of drug therapies with proven benefit. In addition, interventional treatments with coronary artery bypass grafting and percutaneous coronary angioplasty, have prognostic benefit for certain categories of patients. In contrast, non-pharmacological treatments, chief among which are exercise, dietary modification and lifestyle modification, offer promise, but have been much less easy to evaluate. Many of the components of non-pharmacological treatments are addressed by cardiac rehabilitation programmes, which, in the twenty-first century, should provide individually tailored treatments, bearing in mind the differing coronary risk factors that have brought about the patient's coronary event. In this review, these treatments are discussed, together with the coronary risk factor or factors they are designed to treat or modify. Some treatment modalities are designed, however (or have been claimed), to modify more than one risk factor. In some cases the evidence for one effect is good while that for another is weak. In addition, some strategies, which have worked well in carefully designed small-scale studies, may not have widespread applicability.

Risk factor – physical inactivity; intervention – exercise training

Better to hunt in fields, for health unbought
Than fee the doctor for a nauseous draught.
The wise, for cure, on exercise depend;
God never made his work, for man to mend

John Dryden

Physical inactivity continues to increase in westernised populations and is associated with increasing levels of obesity (Kuczmarski *et al.* 1994). Physical inactivity is itself a risk factor for the development of coronary artery disease (Powell & Pratt 1996; Miller & Paffenbarger 1999).

Experimental evidence

Although a number of studies link physical inactivity with increased risk of coronary artery disease, there are no major primary prevention trials (with the possible exception of the MRFIT study, see below), and in many studies it is possible that subtle degrees of incapacitation due to pre-existing coronary artery disease influenced the level of activity undertaken by the subjects under study. One early attempt to counteract this criticism remains one of the best known studies. Over a period of 22 years Paffenbarger *et al.* (1970) studied San Francisco longshoremen. Longshoremen (stevedores) uniquely performed heavy physical exercise for some time on induction to their occupation and in the study were thus indisputably 'fit' at entry to employment. Subsequently, however, those who continued as cargo handlers (physical energy expenditure > 8,500 kcal per week) had reduced coronary events in comparison with hoist operators, clerks and foremen (physical energy expenditure < 8,500 kcal per week). More recent studies in Finland and in the USA have confirmed Paffenbarger's observations (Ekelund *et al.*1988; Lakka *et al.* 1994).

Animal studies

Multiple studies exist of differing species under a variety of atherogenic stresses. The most relevant observations come from primate studies. Kramsch *et al.* (1981) in Boston carried out one of the best studies in this field in Macaque monkeys. In this study, monkeys fed Purina monkey chow were compared with monkeys fed an isocaloric atherogenic diet, and another group fed the atherogenic diet but exercised on a treadmill. The study period was three years. Non-exercise-conditioned monkeys on the atherogenic diet (serum total cholesterol 15.5 mmol/l) showed ischaemic ECG changes, angiographic changes of coronary artery disease and extensive postmortem coronary atherosclerosis. Control monkeys and exercise monkeys did not show these abnormalities, and increases in HDL-cholesterol and reductions in LDL-cholesterol were induced by exercise.

Pathophysiology

It is clear from the above studies and from others (Rauramaa *et al.* 1984) that modification of plasma lipids by regular physical exercise may directly influence coronary risk. Exercise training (or conditioning), however, induces many other physiological changes. These include haemorrheological effects, reductions in plasma fibrinogen (a potent risk factor for hazard in the secondary prevention arena – Koenig 1998), and reductions in myocardial ischaemia, particularly at submaximal workloads. Recently, Hambrecht *et al.* (2000) have demonstrated that exercise training has important effects on coronary vasomotion. Exercise training in subjects with coronary artery disease attenuated paradoxical coronary vasoconstriction to acetylcholine. But there are few studies of exercise alone as a treatment for coronary artery disease. Most programmes using exercise have also combined it with dietary advice, weight reduction and optimisation of ancillary medication. It is difficult therefore to separate the beneficial effects of exercise from other therapies (Gould *et al.* 1992; Schuler *et al.* 1992; Haskell *et al.* 1994), although some striking results have been observed in well-conducted small-scale studies. The study by Hambrecht and colleagues, using quantitative coronary angiography, is perhaps most analogous to the Kramsch study alluded to above.

Clinical evidence

The largest single trial of exercise and its potential beneficial effects on coronary artery disease patients was the National Exercise and Heart Disease Project, sponsored by the National Heart, Lung, and Blood Institute (NHLBI) in the USA (Shaw 1981). Premature withdrawal of funding compromised the conclusions of this study, which showed trends in favour of an intensive one-year exercise programme compared with 'usual care'. This study, however, was incorporated into both of the two substantial overviews of exercise and cardiac rehabilitation published within a short time of each other (Oldridge *et al.* 1988; O'Connor *et al.* 1989). These analyses independently reached broadly similar conclusions. After approximately three years, the reduction in risk of cardiovascular death following participation in a cardiac rehabilitation programme is of the order of 20–25 per cent. But trials included were performed between 1972 and 1985, and the exercise intervention applied varied widely. Follow-up of more than one year was required for the O'Connor analysis and two years for the Oldridge analysis. Almost all trials recruited exclusively male patients under the age of 65 years.

No further analyses of this type will be forthcoming, or indeed will be helpful. The widespread application of secondary prevention pharmacotherapy with its enormous contribution to the prevention of vascular disease progression will make any further demonstration of the benefits of exercise as a sole intervention unethical, and therefore impractical.

Physical exercise does have an important place in symptom management after myocardial infarction. The 'training effect', whereby the patient can achieve an external workload with reduced heart rate and blood pressure compared with the levels before training, is valuable in clinical practice. Both heart rate and systolic blood pressure are important determinants of myocardial oxygen consumption (Ganz & Braunwald 1997). It follows that patients may achieve a level of external work after exercise training that they cannot achieve without experiencing angina pectoris prior to training. Myocardial function may also be improved after training in cardiac patients, particularly if prolonged and intensive (Ehsani *et al.* 1982). Much of the training effect, however, is due to enhanced oxygen extraction by exercising in the trained muscle groups (increased arteriovenous oxygen difference), and is therefore largely obtained at a reduced overall cardiac output (Clausen 1976). This training effect can be quite potent, comparable in clinical results with anti-anginal therapy (Todd & Ballantyne 1990, 1992).

There are many other studies to indicate that exercise in patients after a cardiac event carries benefits, although, as indicated above, few if any in recent years have focused solely on exercise. Exercise conditioning carries other health benefits. These can be summarised as in Table 2.1 (Smith & Wenger 1999).

Table 2.1 Health benefits of exercise

Evidence of benefit	*Inconsistent or absent benefit*
Exercise tolerance	Body weight
Muscle strength	Blood pressure
Symptoms	Lipids
Cigarette smoking cessation (with counselling)	Return to work
Psychological well-being	Non-fatal re-infarction
Social adjustment and functioning	

Exercise is important lifelong but has particular and attractive benefits for elderly people. Longitudinal studies of the age-related decline in maximal aerobic performance, as assessed by maximal oxygen uptake ($\dot{V}o_{2max}$), indicate that between 60 and 90 years minimal aerobic requirement for survival is reached. Exercise conditioning attenuates this decline (Larson & Bruce 1986). But exercise in older people brings other benefits too, some as apparently mundane as the prevention of disabilities caused by immobility – faecal impaction, incontinence, deep vein thrombosis (Young & Dinan 1994). Exercise also increases safety for older people (Fiatarone *et al.* 1994; Campbell *et al.* 1997). Exercise and its contribution to lipid management are further reviewed below, but its continuation in a lifelong pattern is important. Many exercise benefits are lost with discontinuation (Hardman 1999). Exercise is not 'bankable'.

Exercise in heart failure

Exercise in this group of patients has evolved from complete contraindication – 'rest for the body; rest for the mind; rest for the heart' (Lewis 1942) – to accepted practice (European Heart Failure Training Group 1998). Although there is general agreement on rest for acute heart failure between old and new authorities, patients with chronic left ventricular dysfunction can undergo exercise training safely and show benefit. Improvements in peak oxygen consumption and exercise duration are associated with reduced catecholamine levels and other neuroendocrine responses, and improved heart rate variability. These latter markers are known to be associated with poorer prognosis in heart failure, although the conceptual leap between the observation of more favourable neuroendocrine profiles, and improved prognosis has not been demonstrated in adequately sized trials as yet.

A very large document on cardiac rehabilitation from the US Agency for Health Care Policy and Research endorses the opinions expressed above (Wenger *et al.* 1995). Although this group considered some 900 plus publications prior to making its recommendations, it none the less comprised healthcare professionals whose main focus is cardiac rehabilitation. It is encouraging therefore that an independently constituted group has also endorsed the need for greater physical activity in the maintenance of cardiovascular health and prevention of recurrent disease (NIH Consensus Development Panel 1996).

Despite such endorsements, understandable anxiety exists about the possible adverse effects of exercise. It is a common anecdotal experience that some people die suddenly during exercise, due to coronary artery disease, or sustain a heart attack shortly afterward. This phenomenon is sometimes called 'triggering'. Our current knowledge of acute coronary syndromes and myocardial infarction suggests that frequently this is triggered by rupture of a 'vulnerable' coronary artery plaque, although instantaneous death is more commonly due to arrhythmia (Goodman 1999). During violent isometric exercise, substantial increases in cardiac afterload occur, and direct mechanical stress is imposed on the whole of the central vasculature. The phenomenon of 'triggering' has been explored in both Augsburg, Germany, and Boston, USA (Curfman 1993). Although a substantial amount of debate was engendered by the papers discussed by Curfman (1993) (see Correspondence 1994), the essential message is twofold: (1) exercise can act as a trigger of myocardial infarction and (2) paradoxically perhaps, exercise taken regularly is none the less protective. The worst thing to do is never to exercise, and then to have to do so! Pushing a broken down car, or shovelling snow, is not only fixed in the layman's mind as associated with heart attack, it is also borne out by the evidence.

Risk factor – cigarette smoking; intervention – smoking cessation programmes

> To cease smoking is the easiest thing I ever did. I ought to know because I've done it a thousand times.
>
> Mark Twain (attrib.)

Cigarette smoking is the single largest avoidable environmental and behavioural cause of cardiovascular disease, and of course the cause of several forms of cancer (Bartecchi *et al.* 1994). Its highly addictive nature can be seen in studies carried out in drug addiction clinics, in that opiate addicts generally find it easier to give up heroin than to give up smoking. Interventions to promote smoking cessation have been costed at less than £1,000 per life-year gained, in contrast with over 310 other medical interventions with a median cost of about £17,000 per life-year gained. Smoking is therefore a 'best buy' target for healthcare professionals. Intensive support and nicotine replacement therapy are important components of any serious attempts to help heavy smokers, although even brief but assertive medical advice is helpful. Kottke *et al.* (1988) reviewed the attributes of successful smoking cessation interventions in medical practice. Programmes with multiple advisers in the team, multiple methods of approach, and sustained and regular contacts with clients were the most successful. Fiscal measures are also important (Department of Health 1998). Full details of guidelines can be found elsewhere (Raw *et al.* 1998).

Risk factor – hyperlipidaemia; intervention – lifestyle, dietary and behavioural modification

It's a very odd thing –
As odd as can be –
That whatever Miss T. eats
Turns into Miss T.

Walter de la Mare

Hyperlipidaemia is a misnomer, implying that there is a condition characterised by a definable level of plasma or serum lipids that is attended by increased cardiovascular risk. With the exception of certain rare genetically determined lipid abnormalities, there is a continuous graded risk associated with level of plasma cholesterol, both between populations and within a population (American Heart Association, National Heart, Lung, and Blood Institute 1990). Striking data for benefit have accumulated from therapeutic intervention studies. These have largely been with hydroxymethylglutaryl coenzyme A (HMG Co-A) reductase inhibitors. Is there any evidence for non-pharmacological manipulation of plasma lipids?

In the USA, average serum cholesterol has declined by more than 0.6 mmol/l since the 1960s, and in Scandinavian countries a similar effect has been observed since the 1970s. Despite data from the UK indicating substantial falls in butter consumption since 1975, replaced by polyunsaturated or vegetable oils, and increases in the consumption of reduced fat as compared with full-fat milk, a much smaller change has been observed, and this is not satisfactorily explained (Law 1999). Rigorous dieting can improve cholesterol levels, although generally only of the order of 0.3–0.6 mmol/l. It is noteworthy that, in the Scandinavian 4S trial, although the placebo group was given advice on dietary modification, the run-in levels of cholesterol prior to initiation of randomised therapy showed no difference over several months, and continued without any real change on randomised placebo therapy for five years or more (Scandinavian Simvastatin Survival Study Group 1994). This therefore probably represents the 'real world' of treatment effect (or lack of it) with simple dietary advice alone. A systematic overview of dietary intervention trials indicated that diets equivalent to the American Heart Association Step 2 diet (see below) lowered blood total cholesterol by 6.1 per cent and diets equivalent to the American Heart Association Step 1 schema lowered blood total cholesterol by 3.0 per cent ($p<0.0001$; Tang *et al.* 1998). Efficacy was limited by lack of compliance. Overviews of complex interventions, however, are fraught with statistical problems, and the paper by Tang *et al.* has been criticised for inappropriately excluding trials and for drawing conclusions when statistical testing reveals substantial heterogeneity between studies (Davey Smith & Ebrahim 1998).

In a number of small-scale studies, however, relatively large effects on plasma lipids have been found, and in some cases these have been associated with favourable angiographic changes. In the Lifestyle Heart Trial, Ornish *et al.* (1990) sought to modify risk in a multifactorial manner, although with an approach that eschewed drug therapy in favour of major dietary changes, meditation and relaxation therapy, and moderate physical exercise. Although the study populations were small, changes in LDL-cholesterol were quite striking, and this was associated with improved coronary angiographic appearances. In the dietary component, however, only about 10 per cent of total calories were made up of fat. This intake is very markedly below most dietary levels in the Western World. Current US fat intake is 33 per cent of calories; the National Cholesterol Education Program recommends 30 per cent (Step I) and 20 per cent (Step II) (Fair 1999). Dramatic changes in fat intake as in the Lifestyle Heart Trial require very careful dietary planning. This study is surely unique in crediting six chefs for a total treatment population of 48 subjects! Another study incorporating diet in the management of coronary artery disease was the St Thomas' Atherosclerosis Regression Study (STARS). Although an examination of cholestyramine added to dietary treatment, the diet-alone group, in whom the primary aim was to reduce fat intake to 27 per cent of dietary energy, also showed significant falls in LDL-cholesterol compared with a control group over 39 months. Triglyceride levels were also reduced. The dietary strategy also increased intake of omega-3 and omega-6 fatty acids. Plant-derived soluble fibre was also added. Weight did not change significantly. In addition to encouraging results obtained in plasma lipids, improved angiographic appearances were seen in patients treated with diet alone or diet plus cholestyramine in this study (Watts *et al.* 1992).

The STARS study gives a clue to what is perhaps an important feature of successful dietary intervention studies. Not only may it be important to reduce saturated fat intake, it might also be necessary to modify the composition of the ingested fats. A number of studies have examined this possibility. In the DASH study, the effect of dietary patterns on blood pressure was examined (Appel *et al.* 1997). A diet rich in fruits, vegetables, and low-fat dairy products reduced blood pressure more than a control diet in 459 subjects with mild hypertension, independent of sodium or caloric intake. Similarly, in the Lyon Diet Heart Study, after approximately four years in a post-myocardial population, a 'Mediterranean' diet resulted in reduced cardiac events compared with control diet, although the numbers were relatively small (de Lorgeril *et al.* 1999). The Diet And Reinfarction Trial (DART) also modified diet, the most important component being the introduction of fatty fish, with beneficial results (Burr *et al.* 1989). It is notable that modest if any changes in the usual measured plasma lipids occurred in these studies, demonstrating the shortcomings of conventional lipid risk factor measurement. The very substantial GISSI-Prevenzione trial, in 11,324 post-myocardial infarction subjects in Italy, investigated the addition of vitamin E and/or *n*-3 polyunsaturated fatty acids (PUFAs) to the diet. Dietary supplementation with *n*-3 PUFAs led to reduction in death or cardiac events by 10–20 per cent (GISSI-Prevenzione Investigators 1999). There is some evidence that the effects of *n*-3 (ω-3 or omega-3) fatty acids may be mediated by an electrophysiological effect in suppressing malignant ventricular arrhythmias (O'Keefe & Harris 2000). Finally, and most recently, a report from US women in the Breast Cancer Detection and Demonstration Project (BCDDP) indicated that women with a better recommended food score (RFS) have a lower than expected all-cause mortality, despite adjustment for confounding reductions in known coronary risk factors. Although not a clinical trial, this study is powerful because of the large number of events recorded (2,065 deaths after a median follow-up of 5.6 years) from a total of 42,554 women who completed a food frequency questionnaire (Kant *et al.* 2000). The contrasting results of trials of saturated fat reduction and trials where intake of unsaturated fats has been the aim have been reviewed by Oliver (1997).

Other multifactorial intervention studies

Schuler *et al.* (1992) performed a randomised multifactorial intervention trial with an intensive physical exercise programme and a low-fat diet in 113 patients with coronary artery disease. They used the American Heart Association Phase 3 diet with fat intake < 20 per cent of energy. Lipid-lowering drugs were not prescribed. Intensive cardiac investigations were performed at one year of intervention. Coronary artery disease progressed at a slower pace in the intervention group. In the intervention group body weight decreased 5 per cent, total cholesterol by 10 per cent, LDL by 8 per cent and triglycerides by 24 per cent. All changes were highly significant. There are some inconsistencies here with regard to triglyceride levels, which fell in some studies, but failed to do so in others. This issue is partly addressed by Lavie and Milani (1994). In 313 patients not taking any lipid-modifying therapy undertaking an exercise programme and an American Heart Association Phase I diet (National Cholesterol Education Program Expert Panel on Detection, Evaluation, and Treatment of High Blood Cholesterol in Adults 1988) the reductions seen in triglyceride levels were restricted to patients with high baseline triglycerides. This could, however, be an example in part of regression toward the mean.

Some studies (including some very large-scale studies) have failed to show benefit from lifestyle modification (or multifactorial intervention). The best known of these is the Multiple Risk Factor Intervention Trial (MRFIT). In 12,866 high-risk men, changes in diet and adoption of a healthier lifestyle probably occurred in both the special intervention and the usual care group, and cholesterol change was a modest 5 per cent reduction. When one considers that 316,099 white men were screened for this study, and that the lipid changes were so modest, it is scarcely remarkable that attention in the last decade has focused on drugs that can achieve up to 40 per cent lowering of cholesterol, and that can be studied in a double-blinded manner (Blackburn & Leon 1986; Neaton & Wentworth 1992).

Exercise training

Does exercise training itself modify lipoprotein levels in cardiac patients, independent of effects on weight? Tran and Brammell (1989) addressed this question in a meta-analysis. The authors concluded that there were significant trends in favour of lower triglycerides and LDL-cholesterol levels, and increases in HDL-cholesterol levels when the 15 studies examined were pooled. Only five of the fifteen studies, however, had a control group. Weight, of course, could not be controlled in these studies, and when change in cholesterol was measured against change in body weight there was a highly significant relationship (lower weight, lower cholesterol). The data are therefore somewhat flawed but possibly point to a beneficial rather than a deleterious effect of exercise on serum lipids, and are consistent with the animal studies.

It remains likely that diet is important – particularly to the majority of the population who in the long term have a risk of coronary heart disease of about 40 per cent, and yet will not for the most part be taking lipid-lowering drugs. At present, it has been estimated that patients who already have coronary artery disease, but who only have angina, are too costly to treat with statins because the cost–benefit analysis indicates that the drugs are too expensive in terms of quality of life-years gained (Pharoah & Hollingworth 1996). As indicated in the introduction above, dietary manipulations, and spontaneous changes in population diet, will continue and will probably be of benefit in both primary and secondary prevention. In terms of national policy, the North Karelia Project in Finland has continued since 1972 to influence cardiovascular risk in a population of northeast Finland that once had the highest incidence of coronary artery disease in the world. Dramatic changes in the use of fat products have occurred, and there has been a decline in coronary heart disease mortality from about 700 per 100,000 (age-adjusted) to less than 200 per 100,000 in the group of men aged 35–64 years (Puska 1999). The reduction in population cholesterol explains about half of this decline (Vartiainen *et al.* 1994).

Phytosterols in the diet

More aggressive approaches to dietary modification are around the corner. Chisholm *et al.* (1996) studied the effect of replacing butter with margarine of canola (rapeseed like) oil. Concentrations of LDL-cholesterol fell by about 10 per cent. No adverse lipoprotein patterns were found. Novel approaches have been taken with the introduction of proprietary brands of margarine containing plant stanol esters. Plant stanol esters reduce cholesterol absorption and when incorporated into diets low in saturated fat and cholesterol have achieved reductions in LDL-cholesterol of up to 24 per cent (Cater 1999). Finally, changes in the diet of animals can in turn modify the body composition of those animals. This approach has been applied to egg production and to some meats. When consumed by humans, these products appear to have the same beneficial effects as when the original plant fatty acids are eaten. Although entire populations have been treated with plant sterols (in Finland) it remains possible that adverse effects may occur in the long term. Phytosterols, as these compounds are called, are remarkably similar to human sterols, and could potentially interact with steroid hormone biosynthesis (Moghadasian & Frohlich 1999).

Antioxidant vitamins

Considerable interest has been shown in dietary supplementation, particularly with antioxidant vitamins. Although oxygen is essential for life it has been known for many years that excess oxygen has harmful effects. Oxidation of intrinsic structural molecules in the body may result in irreversible change, and there are numerous enzyme systems, which protect against oxidation. It has been hypothesised that LDL-cholesterol, when oxidised, is particularly atherogenic, and that antioxidant vitamins might protect against this (Steinberg *et al.* 1989). Preliminary studies using α-tocopherol and β-carotene have been disappointing (Hennekens *et al.* 1994); although one study using vitamin E supplementation gave positive results, neither the GISSI-Prevenzione trial, nor the recent very large HOPE study, showed any benefit in patients at high risk for coronary artery disease events (GISSI-Prevenzione Investigators 1999; Heart Outcomes Prevention Evaluation Study Investigators 2000). The National Academy of Sciences Institute of Medicine has recently re-evaluated the dietary reference intakes (DRIs) for antioxidant vitamins, selenium and carotenoids, and concluded that definite upper intake levels for these compounds exist, with lack of benefit for pharmacological levels of supplementation (Standing Committee on the Scientific Evaluation of Dietary Reference Intakes [DRIs] 2000).

Other key components of diet have also received attention. One of these is alcohol. Another is chocolate.

Alcohol

High levels of alcohol ingestion are directly damaging to myocardium, possibly through a mechanism involving the non-oxidative metabolism of ethanol to fatty acid ethyl esters (Beckemeier & Bora 1998). In contrast, moderate alcohol consumption is associated with a lower risk of coronary heart disease (Maclure 1993). Although there are potentially confounding reasons for this (in some westernised countries higher alcohol intake is associated with greater wealth and higher socioeconomic status), there is a plausible biological mechanism. Alcohol increases the serum concentration of HDL-cholesterol. The effect does not appear to be specific for any type of alcoholic beverage (Rimm *et al.* 1996). It is unclear how much of the effect relates to the ethanol itself, or to congeners in alcoholic drinks, which have other potentially beneficial effects such as antioxidant activity. One interesting study from Copenhagen indicates that the association between alcohol ingestion and risk of an ischaemic heart disease event is highly dependent on concentration of LDL-cholesterol. In other words, those with the highest baseline risk (high LDL-cholesterol) benefit more from the effect of alcohol than those with lower LDL-cholesterol concentrations (Hein *et al.* 1996).

Chocolate

Chocolate products are obtained by the absorption of natural cocoa solids into the natural oils of the cocoa bean itself (cocoa butter), although substantial adulteration of this material results in many of the products marketed as chocolate. It has been known for many years that the natural product contains antioxidants, which are powerful enough to prevent the rancidification of the fat in chocolate (Waterhouse *et al.* 1996). These properties of chocolate were exploited during the Second World War. US troops were rationed to three chocolate bars per day as their sole source of nourishment during heavy combat. Reports by Waterhouse *et al.* (1996) and Kondo *et al.* (1996) indicate that cocoa can reduce the oxidation of LDL-cholesterol. This property derives from cocoa polyphenols (or flavonoids) such as (–)epicatechin. Whether this property of cocoa is of any significant population benefit is debatable, particularly as so many chocolate products contain substantial amounts of added fat and sugar (see 'obesity' below).

National dietary policies

Many westernised countries have produced proposals for a healthier diet. These policies tend to rely on education and encouragement. What would happen if governments deliberately manipulated our diet by fiscal means? Marshall (2000) has discussed this possibility. His conclusions are challenged by an accompanying paper (Kennedy & Offut 2000). When one examines the improvements in diet over recent years, however, fiscal intervention is not the explanation. Some of the improvement results from changes in farming methods (e.g. the battery rearing of chickens). Some result from greater availability of healthy foods (e.g. the year-round availability of vegetables and fruits brought about by newer cultivation methods and better transport). Some result from the realisation by manufacturers and supermarkets that a 'healthy' label may contribute to higher sales of certain products. Taxation on foodstuffs is not a popular issue.

Risk factor – obesity; intervention – weight reduction

Some of us are out of breath, and all of us are fat!

Lewis Carroll, *Alice through the Looking Glass.*

Western populations continue to increase in weight. In the USA the last decade of the twentieth century saw the prevalence of obesity rise to one-third of the population. In the 1997 *Health Survey for England* (Prescott-Clarke & Primatesta 1999), it was reported that 17 per cent of men and 20 per cent of women in the UK were obese. Obesity correlates with higher mortality and a higher incidence of chronic disease. Concerns have been raised, however, about the risks of losing weight, particularly rapidly, and then often regaining it. Dattilo (1999) has reviewed 70 studies on almost 1,300 subjects and concluded that per kilogram excess weight loss the total cholesterol falls by 0.05 mmol/l, and that favourable influences are seen on glycaemic control in diabetes, lipid oxidisability status, haemostatic factors, left ventricular hypertrophy and blood pressure. Care should be taken to ensure that there is not just substitution of carbohydrate for fat. When study subjects are fed isocaloric diets in which the fat has been substituted by carbohydrate, serum triglycerides tend to increase, and HDL-cholesterol levels tend to decrease (Clinical Debate 1997). Where weight reduction accompanies changes in the energy source in the diet, any adverse changes appear to be lost. One of the clearest indications of the beneficial effects of weight reduction within a single trial is seen in the correlation observed in the MRFIT trial. Weight reduction showed a clear graded relation with total cholesterol reduction (Blackburn & Leon 1986). Control of obesity in itself has not been shown to lower morbidity or mortality in cardiac patients, although the changes above clearly reduce risk, and reduction of excess body fat improves symptoms and lessens fatigue (Squires *et al.* 1990).

Risk factor – stress and psychological causes or modifiers of coronary artery disease; intervention – psychosocial and other forms of behavioural therapy

Most patients (and indeed relatives of patients) when interviewed attribute their coronary artery disease event to stress. There is some evidence to support this view, in terms, for example, of accumulation of stressful events such as divorce, bereavement or unemployment (Blumenthal 1985). Once coronary artery disease is established there is firm evidence to indicate that stress is deleterious and may provoke ischaemic events (Gullette *et al.* 1997; Steptoe 1999). The most well-recognised psychological component of coronary artery disease risk is type A behaviour. The type A personality is hard-driving, competitive, aggressive and impatient. Following a number of studies with null findings in respect of this personality overall, adherents of type A behaviour as a coronary risk factor have pursued the possibility that the hostility element of such behaviour is the most dangerous, in that it promotes rebellion against advice, and continuation of adverse lifestyle traits such as cigarette smoking. The assessment of true type A personality is a skilled task, however (Blumenthal 1985). Modification of lifelong behaviour patterns is difficult, but there is some evidence that a programme of stress management incorporated within a cardiac rehabilitation programme may be beneficial (Blumenthal *et al.* 1997). It is important to realise that, although type A behaviour may be a risk factor for coronary artery disease, once the disease is present, type A personality may predict a better survival, at least for some categories of patients who are at the highest risk. This paradox probably stems from the 'driven' characteristic of such patients, which may improve their adherence to treatment regimens (Barefoot *et al.* 1989). Exercise training in itself does not appear to influence psychosocial functioning, although depressed patients improve (Blumenthal *et al.* 1988). The literature on psychosocial interventions is extremely confused with passionately held views on all sides. A useful overview of cardiac rehabilitation, published by the NHS Centre for Reviews and Dissemination, University of York, discusses this issue (Effective Health Care 1998). Drawing the threads of multiple papers together, it would appear that psychosocial and educational intervention might correct potentially harmful misconceptions about cardiac disease, improve compliance with recommended regimens such as non-smoking, dietary modification and increased physical activity. It appears particularly important to include both patient and spouse or partner. Steptoe (1999) has stated: 'The recognition that an individual's circumstances and personality interact with biological risk factors may provide new opportunities for prevention, and for more refined risk stratification.'

Depression is a manifestation of the most adverse psychosocial reaction to myocardial infarction. In some patients, of course, depression is present beforehand. It is common, with 13–19 per cent of patients exhibiting some features of the disorder. Importantly it is correlated with substantially increased risk of mortality, angina, arrhythmias, rehospitalisation, prolonged disability and continued smoking (Creed 1999).

Studies of rehabilitation in depressed patients probably suffer from the dilution of patients with major problems by patients who form the mass of people suffering from, and then recovering from, any major medical disorder. In addition, the interventions applied to the mass of recovering myocardial infarction patients may not be intensive enough or suited to significantly depressed patients (Barr Taylor *et al.* 1986). Although the major adverse impact on prognosis of significant depression is well documented by Creed (1999), the evidence for benefit is not persuasive – at least in terms of subsequent cardiac morbidity. There can be few, however, who would deny patients adequate care when as many as one in six post-myocardial infarction patients are affected, and specialised help is available, and perhaps too rarely sought.

Other specific problems

Return to work

It is a major failing of pharmacological and particularly surgical therapy for coronary artery disease that, despite evidence of symptomatic and mortality benefit, it does not appear to enhance the recovery of the patient to the extent that he or she returns to work. Most studies have focused on male patients because the numbers are greater, and because the older age of most female patients at presentation with coronary artery disease renders them less likely to be in employment. The factors that predict failure to return to work are well documented. These include: lower achieved level of education, higher physical activity associated with the employment, the severity of the index myocardial infarct and the subjective perception of health status. Other factors such as lack of financial incentives, low socioeconomic status and low personal control over the work performed may also play a part (Smith & O'Rourke 1988). Although more than 70 per cent of patients in some samples return to work after myocardial infarction, the economic costs of the failure to return of the other subjects is very large.

One factor that is important in the UK is duration of sick leave prior to intervention, consistently identified in studies as predicting higher likelihood of failure to return to work following coronary artery bypass grafting (Pravikoff 1999).

What factors can influence the likelihood that a patient will return to work? One study found that physicians' advice was of vital importance (Usher *et al.* 1986). The overall 'modality' of cardiac rehabilitation does not appear to influence it (Wenger *et al.* 1995). Exercise testing itself, however, has a limited but definite influence on return to work, possibly by virtue of the objective demonstration in the controlled healthcare setting that the preconceived anxieties of the patient are unfounded (Dennis *et al.* 1988). In this study, return to full-time work occurred at a median of 51 days in intervention patients, simple though this intervention was, compared with a median of 75 days in patients receiving usual care.

The decision to return to work includes both 'if' and 'when'. Patients will obviously look to the healthcare professional that they have most contact with to seek advice about both of these issues. The opportunity to influence the patient's decision is obvious and an important responsibility.

Compliance with lifestyle modification behaviour

Observations within and outwith cardiac rehabilitation programmes indicate that important lifestyle interventions are not adhered to long term (Burke 1999). Three specific areas can be identified. These are:

1. Patient-related factors – these can be predicted by the patient's initial adherence, their self-efficacy and social support.
2. Regimen-related factors – a more complex treatment regimen predicts non-adherence.

3. Provider-related factors – these relate to the empathic and communication and motivational skills of the healthcare professional delivering therapy.

As well as exploring the patient's readiness to change behaviour (Prochaska & Congdon 1999) it is important to emphasise the concept of self-efficacy, where the power to change is seen to reside within the patient himself or herself. Other strategies include the involvement of partners, self-monitoring, reinforcement, multiple contacts and goal setting. When lifestyle modification advice is delivered in a cardiac rehabilitation programme, extended-length participation predicts better control of body weight, physical fitness and lipoprotein subfractions, and may be an argument for continuing centre-based programmes (Brubaker *et al.* 1996). Lack of funding and other practical issues suggest, however, that strategies for enhancing adherence to home-exercise and dietary programmes will be needed.

Cardiac rehabilitation – the 'package'

It is possible that much of the very substantial improvement documented by Oldridge *et al.* (1988) and O'Connor *et al.* (1989) in cardiovascular mortality after myocardial infarction mediated by cardiac rehabilitation was due to improved surveillance of cardiac patients and better application of therapy. The only therapies available to most of the programmes in the 1970s and early 1980s were first β blockade, and second aspirin, although perhaps better control of blood pressure with therapy could also have played a part. We will never know how much, if any, of the treatment benefit was mediated by the lifestyle modifications discussed above.

The evidence that a variety of strategies discussed above may modify patient risk over and above the powerful armamentarium of the pharmacopoeia is compelling when viewed in totality, and cardiac rehabilitation programmes are well placed to begin to help the patient presenting with coronary artery disease, although home-based programmes and strategies for transferring the process of care smoothly, and still effectively, to the primary care sector continue to be assessed. In this regard, one factor that is as yet often not alluded to or admitted is the skills, knowledge base, and motivational ability of the member of the team delivering the message to the patient. 'There is no fancy facility nor exciting piece of equipment that can ensure patient compliance better than excellent staff' (Hall 1999).

Despite weaknesses highlighted throughout this review in the evidence base, it is clear that responsible and objective scientists feel that cardiac rehabilitation has a role to play in the management of patients with coronary artery disease, over and above merely enhancing adherence to drug treatment regimens. The conclusions of the executive summary of the US Agency for Health Care Policy and Research (AHCPR) state: 'On the basis of a comprehensive review of the scientific literature, the panel concludes that cardiac rehabilitation services are an essential component of the contemporary management of patients with multiple presentations of CHD and with heart failure. Cardiac rehabilitation is a multifactorial process that includes exercise training, education, counseling regarding risk reduction and lifestyle changes, and use of behavioural interventions; these services should be integrated into the comprehensive care of cardiac patients. The objective of cardiac rehabilitation services is to improve both the physiologic and psychosocial status of cardiac patients. The physiologic outcomes targeted include improvement in exercise capacity and exercise habits and optimization of risk-factor status, including improvement in blood lipid and lipoprotein profiles, body weight, and blood glucose and blood pressure levels, and the cessation of smoking. Enhancements of myocardial perfusion and performance, as well as reduction in progression of the underlying atherosclerotic process, are additional goals. The psychosocial functioning of patients should be improved when needed, including reduction of stress, anxiety, and depression. Functional independence of patients, particularly the elderly, is an essential goal of cardiac rehabilitation services. Return to appropriate and satisfactory work could benefit both patients and society' (Wenger *et al.* 1995).

Acknowledgements

I would like to thank my wife Lindsay for putting up with the necessary hours required to put this review together, and an unknown adult education teacher in North Carolina for teaching me to type.

References

American Heart Association, National Heart, Lung, and Blood Institute (1990). The cholesterol facts: a summary of the evidence relating dietary fats, serum cholesterol, and coronary heart disease. *Circulation* **81**, 1721–133

Appel LJ *et al.* (1997). A clinical trial of the effects of dietary patterns on blood pressure. *New England Journal of Medicine* **336**, 1117–1124

Barefoot JC *et al.* (1989). Type A behavior and survival: a follow-up study of 1,467 patients with coronary artery disease. *American Journal of Cardiology* **64**, 427–432

Barr Taylor C *et al.* (1986). The effects of exercise training programs on psychosocial improvement in uncomplicated postmyocardial infarction patients. *Journal of Psychosomatic Research* **30**, 581–587

Bartecchi CE *et al.* (1994). The human costs of tobacco use (Part 1). *New England Journal of Medicine* **330**, 907–912

Beckemeier ME & Bora PS (1998). Fatty acid ethyl esters: potentially toxic products of myocardial ethanol metabolism. *Journal of Molecular and Cellular Cardiology* **30**, 2487–2494

Blackburn H & Leon AS (1986). Preventive cardiology in practice: Minnesota studies on risk factor reduction. In: Pollock ML & Schmidt DH (eds), *Heart Disease and Rehabilitation, Second Edition.* New York: John Wiley & Sons, pp. 265–301

Blumenthal JA (1985). Psychologic assessment in cardiac rehabilitation. *Journal of Cardiopulmonary Rehabilitation* **5**, 208–215

Blumenthal JA *et al.* (1988). The effects of exercise training on psychosocial functioning after myocardial infarction. *Journal of Cardiopulmonary Rehabilitation* **8**, 183–193

Blumenthal JA *et al.* (1997). Stress management and exercise training in cardiac patients with myocardial ischaemia. *Archives of Internal Medicine* **157**, 2213–2223

Brubaker PH *et al.* (1996). Comparison of standard- and extended-length participation in cardiac rehabilitation on body composition, functional capacity and blood lipids. *American Journal of Cardiology* **78**, 769–773

Burke LE (1999). Adherence to a heart-healthy lifestyle – what makes the difference? In Wenger NK *et al.* (eds). *Cardiac Rehabilitation. A Guide to Practice in the 21st Century*. Basel: Marcel Dekker, Inc, pp. 385–393

Burr ML *et al.* (1989). Effects of changes in fat, fish, and fibre intakes on death and myocardial infarction: Diet and Reinfarction Trial (DART). *The Lancet* **ii**, 757–761

Campbell AJ *et al.* (1997). Randomised controlled trial of a general practice programme of home based exercise to prevent falls in elderly women. *British Medical Journal* **315**, 1065–1069

Cater NB (1999). Historical and scientific basis for the development of plant stanol ester foods as cholesterol-lowering agents. *European Heart Journal Supplements* **1**, S36–S44

Chisholm A *et al.* (1996). Effect on lipoprotein profile of replacing butter with margarine in a low fat diet: randomised crossover study with hypercholesterolaemic subjects. *British Medical Journal* **312**, 931–934

Clausen JP (1976). Circulatory adjustments to dynamic exercise and effect of physical training in normal subjects and in patients with coronary artery disease. *Progress in Cardiovascular Disease* **18**, 459–495

Clinical Debate (1997). Should a low-fat, high-carbohydrate diet be recommended for everyone? *New England Journal of Medicine* **337**, 562–567

Correspondence (1994). Triggering of acute myocardial infarction by exercise. *New England Journal of Medicine* **330**, 1156–1157

Creed F (1999). The importance of depression following myocardial infarction. *Heart* **82**, 406–408

Curfman GD (1993). Is exercise beneficial – or hazardous – to your heart? *New England Journal of Medicine* **329**, 1730–1731

Dattilo A (1999). Weight management and exercise in the treatment of obesity. In Wenger NK *et al.* (eds). *Cardiac Rehabilitation. A Guide to Practice in the 21st Century.* Basel: Marcel Dekker, Inc., pp. 247–256

Davey Smith G & Ebrahim S (1998). Commentary: Dietary change, cholesterol reduction, and the public health – what does meta-analysis add? *British Medical Journal* **316**, 1220

De Lorgeril M *et al.* (1999). Mediterranean diet, traditional risk factors, and the rate of cardiovascular complications after myocardial infarction. final report of the Lyon Diet Heart Study. *Circulation* **99**, 779–785

Dennis *et al.* (1988). Early return to work after uncomplicated myocardial infarction. Results of a randomized trial. *Journal of the American Medical Association* **260**, 214–220

Department of Health (1998). *Smoking Kills. A White Paper on Tobacco.* London: Stationery Office

Effective Health Care (1998). *Cardiac Rehabilitation,* Vol 4. Plymouth: Latimer Trend & Co. Ltd, pp 1–12

Ehsani A *et al.* (1982). Cardiac effects of prolonged and intense training in patients with coronary artery disease. *American Journal of Cardiology* **50**, 246–254

Ekelund L-G *et al.* (1988). Physical fitness as a predictor of cardiovascular mortality in asymptomatic north American men. The Lipid Research Clinics Mortality Follow-up Study. *New England Journal of Medicine* **319**, 1379–1384

European Heart Failure Training Group (1998). Experience from controlled trials of physical training in chronic heart failure. Protocol and patient factors in effectiveness in the improvement in exercise tolerance. *European Heart Journal* **19**, 466–475

Fair JM (1999). Lipid lowering for coronary risk reduction. In Wenger NK *et al.* (eds), *Cardiac Rehabilitation. A Guide to Practice in the 21st Century*. Basel: Marcel Dekker, Inc., pp. 223–233

Fiatarone MA *et al.* (1994). Exercise training and nutritional supplementation for physical frailty in very elderly people. *New England Journal of Medicine* **330**, 1769–1775

Ganz P & Braunwald E (1997). Coronary blood flow and myocardial ischaemia. In Braunwald E (ed.), *Heart Disease. A Textbook of Cardiovascular Medicine,* 5th edn. Philadelphia: WB Saunders Co., pp. 1161–1163

GISSI-Prevenzione Investigators (Gruppo Italiano per lo Studio della Sopravivenza nell' infarto miocardico) (1999). Dietary supplementation with n-3 polyunsaturated fatty acids and vitamin E after myocardial infarction: results of the GISSI-Prevenzione trial. *The Lancet* **354**, 447–455

Goodman JM (1999). Sudden cardiac death and exercise in healthy adults. In Shephard RJ & Miller HS Jr (eds), *Exercise and the Heart in Health and Disease*. Basel: Marcel Dekker, Inc., pp. 303–318

Gould KL *et al.* (1992). Improved stenosis geometry by quantitative coronary arteriography after vigorous risk factor modification. *American Journal of Cardiology* **69**, 845–853

Gullette EC *et al.* (1997). Effects of mental stress on left ventricular and peripheral vascular performance in patients with coronary artery disease. *Journal of the American Medical Association* **277**, 1521–1526

Hall LK (1999). Life-long exercise: counseling for exercise maintenance. In Wenger NK *et al.* (eds), *Cardiac Rehabilitation. A Guide to Practice in the 21st Century.* Basel: Marcel Dekker, Inc., pp. 95–101

Hambrecht R *et al.* (1993). Various intensities of leisure time physical activity in patients with coronary artery disease: effects on cardiorespiratory fitness and progression of coronary atherosclerotic lesions. *Journal of the American College of Cardiology* **22**, 468–477

Hambrecht R *et al.* (2000). Effect of exercise on coronary endothelial function in patients with coronary artery disease. *New England Journal of Medicine* **342**, 454–460

Hardman AE (1999). Role of exercise and weight loss in maximizing LDL cholesterol reduction. *European Heart Journal Supplements* **1**, S123–S131

Haskell WL *et al.* (1994). Effects of intensive multiple risk factor reduction on coronary atherosclerosis and clinical cardiac events in men and women with coronary artery disease. The Stanford Coronary Risk Intervention Project (SCRIP). *Circulation* **89**, 975–990

Hein HO *et al.* (1996). Alcohol consumption, serum low density lipoprotein cholesterol concentration, and risk of ischaemic heart disease: six year follow up in the Copenhagen male study. *British Medical Journal* **312**, 736–741

Hennekens CH *et al.* (1994). Antioxidant vitamins – benefits not yet proved. *New England Journal of Medicine* **330**, 1080–1081

Kant AK *et al.* (2000). A prospective study of diet quality and mortality in women. *Journal of the American Medical Association* **283**, 2109–2115

Kennedy E & Offut S (2000). Commentary: alternative nutrition outcomes using a fiscal food policy. *British Medical Journal* **320**, 304–305

Koenig W (1998). Haemostatic risk factors for cardiovascular diseases. *European Heart Journal* **19**, C39–C43

Kondo K *et al.* (1996). Inhibition of LDL oxidation by cocoa. *The Lancet* **348**, 1514

Kramsch DM *et al.* (1981). Reduction of coronary atherosclerosis by moderate conditioning exercise in monkeys on an atherogenic diet. *New England Journal of Medicine* **305**, 1483–1489

Kuczmarski RJ *et al.* (1994). Increasing prevalence of overweight among US adults: the National Health and Nutrition Examination Surveys, 1960–1991. *Journal of the American Medical Association* **272**, 205–211

Lakka TA *et al.* (1994). Relation of leisure-time physical activity and cardiorespiratory fitness to the risk of acute myocardial infarction in men. *New England Journal of Medicine* **330**, 1549–1554

Larson EB & Bruce RA (1986). Exercise and aging. *Annals of Internal Medicine* **106,** 783–785

Lavie CJ & Milani RV (1994). Effects of cardiac rehabilitation and exercise training on low-density lipoprotein cholesterol in patients with hypertriglyceridemia and coronary artery disease. *American Journal of Cardiology* **74**, 1192–1195

Law MR (1999). Lowering heart disease risk with cholesterol reduction: evidence from observational studies and clinical trials. *European Heart Journal Supplements* **1**, S3–S8

Lewis T (1942). *Diseases of the Heart.* London: Macmillan & Co. Ltd.

Maclure M (1993). Demonstration of deductive meta-analysis: ethanol intake and risk of myocardial infarction. *Epidemiology Reviews* **15**, 328–351

Marshall T (2000). Exploring a fiscal food policy: the case of diet and ischaemic heart disease. *British Medical Journal* **320**, 301–304

Miller HS Jr & Paffenbarger RS Jr (1999). The prevention and treatment of coronary disease: the case for exercise. In Shephard RJ & Miller HS Jr (eds), *Exercise and the Heart in Health and Disease,* 2nd edn. Basel: Marcel Dekker, Inc., pp. 295–301

Moghadasian MH & Frohlich JJ (1999). Effects of dietary phytosterols on cholesterol metabolism and atherosclerosis: clinical and experimental evidence. *American Journal of Medicine* **107**, 588–594

National Cholesterol Education Program (1988). Expert Panel on detection, evaluation, and treatment of high blood cholesterol in adults. *Archives of Internal Medicine* **148**, 36–69

Neaton JD & Wentworth D for the Multiple risk Factor Intervention Group (1992). Serum cholesterol, blood pressure, cigarette smoking and death from coronary heart disease: overall findings and differences by age for 316,099 white men. *Archives of Internal Medicine* **152**, 56–64

NIH Consensus Development Panel (1996). Physical activity and cardiovascular health. *Journal of the American Medical Association* **276**, 241–246

O'Connor GT *et al.* (1989). An overview of randomized clinical trials of rehabilitation with exercise after myocardial infarction. *Circulation* **80**, 234–244

O'Keefe JH & Harris WS (2000). Omega-3 fatty acids: time for clinical implementation? *American Journal of Cardiology* **85**, 1239–1241

Oldridge N *et al.* (1988). Cardiac rehabilitation after myocardial infarction: combined experience of randomized clinical trials. *Journal of the American Medical Association* **260**, 945–950

Oliver MF (1997). It is more important to increase the intake of unsaturated fats than to decrease the intake of saturated fats: evidence from clinical trials relating to ischemic heart disease. *American Journal of Clinical Nutrition* **66**, 980S–986S

Ornish D *et al.* (1990). Can lifestyle changes reverse coronary heart disease? *The Lancet* **336**, 129–133

Paffenbarger RS *et al.* (1970). Work activity of longshoremen as related to death from coronary heart disease and stroke. *New England Journal of Medicine* **282**, 1109–1114

Pharoah PDP & Hollingworth (1996). Cost effectiveness of lowering cholesterol concentration with statins in patients with and without pre-existing coronary heart disease: life table method applied to health authority population. *British Medical Journal* **312**, 1443–1448

Powell KE & Pratt M (1996). Physical activity and health. *British Medical Journal* **313**, 126–127

Prescott-Clarke P& Primatesta P (1999). *Health Survey for England 1997.* London: HMSO

Prochaska JO & Congdon K (1999). In Wenger NK *et al.* (eds), *Cardiac Rehabilitation. A Guide to Practice in the 21st Century.* Basel: Marcel Dekker, Inc., pp. 361–370

Puska P (1999). The North Karelia Project: from community intervention to national activity in lowering cholesterol levels and CHD risk. *European Heart Journal Supplements* **1**, S9–S13

Pravikoff DS (1999). Return to work: factors and issues of vocational counselling. In Wenger NK *et al.* (eds), *Cardiac Rehabilitation. A Guide to Practice in the 21st Century.* Basel: Marcel Dekker, Inc., pp. 295–302

Rauramaa R *et al.* (1984). Effects of mild physical exercise on serum lipoproteins and metabolites of arachidonic acid: a controlled randomised trial in middle aged men. *British Medical Journal* **288**, 603–606

Raw M *et al.* (1998). Smoking cessation guidelines for health professionals. A guide to effective smoking cessation interventions for the health care system. *Thorax* **53**, S1–S19

Rimm EB *et al.* (1996). Review of moderate alcohol consumption and reduced risk of coronary heart disease: is the effect due to beer, wine, or spirits? *British Medical Journal* **312**, 731–736

Scandinavian Simvastatin Survival Study Group (1994). Randomised trial of cholesterol lowering in 4444 patients with coronary heart disease. *The Lancet* **344**, 1383–9

Schuler G *et al.* (1992). Regular physical exercise and low-fat diet. Effects on progression of coronary artery disease. *Circulation* **86**, 1–11

Shaw LW (1981). Effects of a prescribed supervised exercise program on mortality and cardiovascular morbidity in patients after myocardial infarction: the National Exercise and Heart Disease Project. *American Journal of Cardiology* **48**, 39–46

Smith GR Jr & O'Rourke DF (1988). Return to work after a first myocardial infarction. A test of multiple hypotheses. *Journal of the American Medical Association* **259**, 1673–1677

Smith LK & Wenger NK (1999). Benefits of exercise training. In Wenger NK *et al.* (eds), *Cardiac Rehabilitation. A Guide to Practice in the 21st Century*. Basel: Marcel Dekker, Inc., pp. 9–18

Squires RW *et al.* (1990). Cardiovascular rehabilitation: status 1990. *Mayo Clinic Proceedings* **65**, 731–755

Standing Committee on the Scientific Evaluation of Dietary Reference Intakes (DRIs). (2000). *Dietary Reference Intakes for Vitamin C, Vitamin E, Selenium, and Carotenoids.* Washington: National Academy Press

Steinberg D *et al.* (1989). Beyond cholesterol: modifications of low-density lipoprotein that increase its atherogenicity. *New England Journal of Medicine* **320**, 915–924

Steptoe A (1999). Psychosocial factors in the aetiology of coronary heart disease. *Heart* **82**, 258–259

Tang JL *et al.* (1998). Systematic review of dietary intervention trials to lower blood total cholesterol in free-living subjects. *British Medical Journal* **316**, 1213–1219

with significantly less progression of atherosclerotic lesions. A surprising finding to emerge from these studies, which were relatively small and short term, was a reduction in clinical events which was significant in some of the individual studies but highly significant when the results of studies were combined in meta-analysis (Brown *et al.* 1993; Superko & Krauss 1994).

Thompson (1997), in a meta-analysis of nine angiographic studies, demonstrated a linear relationship between the change in stenosis diameter and the change in LDL-cholesterol. LDL-cholesterol reduction of approximately 45 per cent was associated with regression.

Major outcome studies

Despite encouraging indications from epidemiology, the early studies and the angiographic studies it was clear that cholesterol lowering would not be introduced into general clinical practice until a definitive clinical trial of cholesterol lowering demonstrated not only a reduction in coronary events but also reductions in overall mortality. This information was provided by the landmark Scandinavian Simvastatin Survival Study (4S) (4S Study Group 1994). This was a randomised, placebo-controlled, multicentre study throughout the Nordic countries involving 4,444 male and female (872) patients aged 35–70 years with established CHD as manifest by a previous myocardial infarction or stable angina (approximately 20 per cent). The fasting total cholesterol concentration at entry was between 5.5 and 8 mmol/l after eight weeks of dietary therapy using the American Heart Association's Step 1 diet. The HMG-CoA reductase inhibitor simvastatin was used at a starting dose of 20 mg daily. In the treatment group, the dose of simvastatin could be increased as necessary to achieve the goal of therapy, a total cholesterol between 3 and 5.2 mmol/l. Of the patients, 37 per cent required an increase to 40 mg daily. Simvastatin therapy was associated with a 35 per cent reduction in LDL-cholesterol, an 8 per cent increase in HDL-cholesterol and a 10 per cent reduction in triglyceride.

The median follow-up time was 5.4 years when the requisite number of deaths (n = 440) had occurred to provide the statistical power to address the primary endpoint of the study, overall mortality. There were 256 deaths in the placebo group and 182 deaths in the simvastatin group, giving a relative risk reduction of 0.7 (95 per cent confidence interval [95%CI] 0.59–0.85; p = 0.0003). In addition to the highly significant reduction in the primary endpoints, secondary endpoints including non-fatal myocardial infarction, coronary death, the need for revascularisation procedures and admissions to hospital were all markedly decreased. A subsequent report showed that the relative risk reduction achieved with simvastatin was similar in those individuals whose LDL-cholesterol was in the lowest quartile at baseline compared to those in the highest quartile (4S Study Group 1995).

The safety analysis of the 4S study was very reassuring in that there were no increases in non-cardiovascular deaths and the overall frequency of adverse events was similar in both the simvastatin and placebo groups. Significant elevations in liver enzymes were seen in only small numbers of patients. Major increases in creatine phosphokinase (more than tenfold) were rare and there was only one case of rhabdomyolysis in a female patient taking 20 mg/day of simvastatin. The patient recovered when the simvastatin was stopped. There were no differences in non-fatal cancer cases between the placebo and simvastatin groups.

The Cholesterol and Recurrent Events (CARE) study (Sacks *et al.* 1996) addressed the question of whether the reduction of an average cholesterol concentration with the HMG-CoA reductase inhibitor pravastatin (40 mg/day) would reduce the risk of coronary events in patients with previous myocardial infarction. The study population consisted of 4,159 male and female (14 per cent) patients aged 21–75 years with previous myocardial infarction. Total cholesterol at entry was below 6.2 mmol/l which corresponded to an LDL-cholesterol of around 3–4.5 mmol/l. In addition to the 'normal' cholesterol the participants in this study were at lower risk because of previous coronary artery bypass grafts or percutaneous transluminal coronary angioplasty (PTCA) in 55 per cent of the participants. In addition, 83 per cent were taking aspirin, 40 per cent β blockers and 39 per cent calcium-channel blockers. The triglyceride entry criteria differed to that of 4S in that a baseline triglyceride concentration of up to 4.4 mmol/l was allowed whereas in the 4S Study the triglyceride baseline had to be < 2.5 mmol/l. Patients with left ventricular dysfunction were allowed in the trial as long as the left ventricular ejection fraction was 25 per cent or more. During the course of the study, LDL-cholesterol was reduced by 28 per cent in the treated group, HDL rose by 5 per cent and triglyceride fell by 14 per cent. The major endpoint of the study was a combination of fatal and non-fatal myocardial infarction, and pravastatin treatment was associated with a 24 per cent reduction (95%CI 9–36; $p = 0.0003$). This study extends potential benefit for cholesterol lowering to post-myocardial infarction survivors with average cholesterol concentrations.

A third major secondary prevention trial, the Longterm Intervention with Pravastatin in Ischaemic Heart Disease study (LIPID), was a large multicentre, randomised, double-masked study performed in Australia and New Zealand (LIPID Study Group, 1998); 9,014 male and female (17 per cent) patients aged 31–75 years were recruited with either a previous history of acute myocardial infraction or hospitalisation for unstable angina 3–36 months previously. They were randomly allocated to pravastatin 40 mg/day or placebo. The entry criterion for total plasma cholesterol was between 4 and 7 mmol/l and plasma triglycerides were allowed up to 5 mmol/l. The primary endpoint of the study was mortality from CHD. At baseline, a substantial numbers of patients were receiving aspirin (82 per cent) and β blockers (47 per cent) and 41 per cent of the patients had undergone revascularisation procedures. Pravastatin therapy produced an LDL-cholesterol reduction of 25 per cent, triglyceride reduction of 11 per cent and a 5 per cent increase in HDL compared with placebo.

In the placebo group, 8.3 per cent of patients died from CHD compared with 6.4 per cent in the pravastatin group, a relative risk reduction of 24 per cent (95%CI 12–35; $p < 0.001$). Overall mortality was also significantly decreased (relative risk reduction 22 per cent, $p < 0.001$) and there was a consistent reduction in all cardiovascular outcomes including myocardial infraction, death from CHD or non-fatal myocardial infarction, and coronary revascularisation. Pravastatin therapy was not associated with clinically significant adverse effects.

It is clear from these trials that there is overwhelming evidence of benefit for cholesterol lowering with statins in individuals with CHD. Subgroup analyses have indicated that older patients and women (Miettinen *et al.* 1997) and people with diabetes (Pyörälä *et al.* 1997; Goldberg *et al.* 1998; Haffner *et al.* 1999) show similar relative risk reductions. A surprising finding in the 4S Study was a 30 per cent reduction in stroke incidence. This was a post-hoc analysis of the data. In CARE there was a preplanned analysis of stroke incidence and, again, approximately a 30 per cent reduction in stroke was observed. In the LIPID trial there were 419 strokes (309 ischaemic) in 373 patients. In the placebo group the risk of stroke was 4.5 per cent compared with 3.7 per cent in the pravastatin group, a relative risk reduction of 19 per cent (95%CI 0–34, $p = 0.05$). This finding was the result of a significant reduction in non-haemorrhagic stroke. There was no difference in haemorrhagic stroke between placebo and pravastatin-treated groups (White *et al.* 2000).

Benefits of intervention to increase HDL-cholesterol

Given that HDL-cholesterol is inversely related to CHD risk, it is important to know whether increasing HDL-cholesterol therapeutically will decrease CHD events. The Veterans Administration HDL Intervention Trial (VA-HIT) was designed to test the potential benefit of therapy to increase HDL-cholesterol in CHD patients where the primary lipid abnormality was a low HDL-cholesterol (Rubins *et al.* 1999). The double-masked trial randomised 2,531 men with established CHD and low HDL-cholesterol (≤ 40 mg/dl; ≤ 1.0 mmol/l) and relatively normal LDL-cholesterol concentration (≤ 140 mg/dl; ≤ 3.6 mmol/l). The therapeutic intervention was the fibric acid derivative gemfibrozil (1,200 mg/day) because this drug increases HDL with little effect on total and LDL-cholesterol. Baseline lipid concentrations were LDL-cholesterol 2.9 mmol/l, HDL-cholesterol 0.8 mmol/l and triglycerides 1.8 mmol/l. At one year, gemfibrozil therapy was associated with no change in LDL-cholesterol but a 6 per cent increase in HDL. Gemfibrozil reduced triglycerides by 31 per cent. The primary outcome measure was the combined incidence of non-fatal myocardial infarction or CHD death. Secondary endpoints included stroke, transient ischaemic attack, revascularisation procedures, carotid endarterectomy, hospitalisation for unstable angina or congestive heart failure, and death from any cause. There were 275 primary events in the placebo group and 219 in the gemfibrozil group, a relative risk reduction of 22 per cent (95%CI 7–35, $p = 0.006$).

For the combined outcome of CHD death, non-fatal myocardial infarction (MI) and stroke there was a 24 per cent reduction ($p < 0.001$).

An interesting subgroup analysis of VA-HIT relates to diabetes. Clinical history identified 627 patients with diabetes. Although caution is necessary because there was a lack of stratification based on diabetes, there was a significant reduction in the combined endpoint (CHD death, non-fatal MI and confirmed stroke) of 24 per cent (95%CI 0.1–43; $p = 0.05$). Although the study hypothesis of VA-HIT was that increasing HDL-cholesterol would benefit outcome, it is clear that this could be the result of other factors, including the reduction of triglyceride, which would also modulate postprandial lipaemia and result in a shift of LDL subfraction distribution to larger more buoyant particles.

A further secondary prevention trial using a fibrate – the Bezafibrate Infarction Prevention (BIP) study – has recently been published (BIP Study Group 2000). In this double-masked, controlled trial, 3,090 (2,825 men) patients with previous myocardial infarction or stable angina were randomised to bezafibrate 400 mg/day or placebo. Lipid entry criteria were total cholesterol of 180–250 mg/dl, LDL-cholesterol ≤ 180 mg/dl, HDL-cholesterol ≤ 45 mg/dl and total triglycerides ≤ 300 mg/dl. Baseline lipid and lipoprotein concentrations were total cholesterol 212 mg/dl, LDL-cholesterol 148 mg/dl, HDL-cholesterol 34.6 mg/dl and total triglycerides 145 mg/dl. In the bezafibrate-treated group the major lipid changes were an increase in HDL-cholesterol of 18 per cent and a reduction of triglycerides by 21 per cent. The primary endpoint of the study was the combination of fatal and non-fatal myocardial infarction or sudden death. The study had a power of between 62 per cent and 85 per cent to detect a 20–25 per cent reduction in CHD incident rate with bezafibrate. After 6.2 years the cumulative probability of the primary endpoint was reduced by 7.3 per cent ($p = 0.24$) with bezafibrate therapy. A post-hoc analysis of patients with high baseline triglycerides (≥ 200 mg/dl) demonstrated a 39.5 per cent ($p = 0.02$) reduction in the primary endpoint. This finding has to be interpreted with caution, however.

Why differing results should be observed in the VA-HIT and BIP studies is open to question as discussed by Haffner (2000). Leaving aside the possibility of inherent differences between the two fibrates, the differences in lipid entry criteria, the smaller number of people with diabetes in BIP and the play of chance could be important. The last is a possibility given that the percentage reduction in events in BIP lies within the confidence intervals observed in VA-HIT.

Mechanisms of benefit of lipid lowering

It is clear from the major lipid-lowering trials that CHD events are reduced effectively and that this reduction is both statistically and clinically significant. This is the main message for clinicians; however, there is no doubt that much will be learned in the future concerning the mechanisms of benefit of these interventions, which should cast new light on the pathological processes involved in the development and progression of atherosclerotic lesions.

It is clear from meta-analyses of the many coronary artery angiographic trials and the more limited trials targeting non-coronary vessels that lipid lowering (primarily LDL-cholesterol lowering) is associated with changes in angiographic parameters. In one such analysis by Thompson (1997), a positive relationship was demonstrated between change in stenosis diameter and the reduction of LDL-cholesterol. When the LDL-cholesterol reduction was greater than 45 per cent, regression was observed. It is likely, however, that these effects observed with computerised techniques of angiographic analysis are insufficient to explain fully the observed effects on clinical events. It is beyond the scope of this chapter to explore in detail the potential mechanisms of benefit. Briefly, stabilisation of the vulnerable plaque (lipid rich with thin fibrous cap) and improved endothelial function are thought to be of importance and are supported by various strands of clinical and experimental evidence.

Guidelines for secondary prevention with lipid-lowering drugs

Given the overwhelming evidence of benefit of cholesterol lowering with statins in these well-conducted, endpoint trials, it is possible to provide clear evidence-based guidelines for lipid-lowering therapy in the patient with established CHD. Furthermore, as atheroma is a generalised disease, these guidelines can be extended to patients who present with disease in other areas such as peripheral vascular disease and carotid artery disease. The joint guidelines of the British societies (British Cardiac Society, British Hyperlipidaemia Association, British Hypertension Society and endorsed by Diabetes UK) provide a detailed, comprehensive review of the evidence for secondary prevention (Wood *et al.* 1998). The threshold for initiating statin treatment suggested is a total cholesterol ≥ 5 mmol/l and/or an LDL-cholesterol ≥ 3.0 mmol/l. The LDL-cholesterol treatment target is suggested as 'at least' an LDL-cholesterol < 3.0 mmol/l. In other guidelines, e.g. the British Hyperlipidaemia Association advice sheet on secondary prevention and the National Cholesterol Education Program in the USA, an LDL goal of < 2.5 mmol/l is suggested. It is recommended that the dose of statin prescribed should be the same as that used in the trials and that an LDL reduction of at least 30 per cent should be sought. A small but important group of patients in whom statins have been shown to be of considerable benefit is the post-cardiac transplant population. Both pravastatin and simvastatin have been shown to improve survival in these patients (Kobashigawa *et al.* 1995; Wenke *et al.* 1997).

Statins will be the first-line agent for the great majority of patients. However, renewed interest in the use of fibrate drugs in certain patients has been rekindled following publication of the VA-HIT. The impact of this study on clinical practice is uncertain. Perhaps in the high-risk individual with an acceptable LDL-cholesterol but a low HDL-cholesterol and hypertriglyceridaemia, a fibrate should be considered. However, in retrospect, a statin comparator in VA-HIT would have been of considerable interest. Although mean baseline LDL-cholesterol was 2.9 mmol/l, which is within the goal as proposed by the joint British societies (<3 mmol/l), many patients would have qualified for statin therapy. As far as the author's practice is concerned the results of the VA-HIT have encouraged more combination therapy. In the high-risk patient established on an effective statin dose with an ideal LDL-cholesterol (the author follows the NCEP guidelines) but a persistent low HDL and raised triglycerides, a fibrate is added. In the author's experience, serious side effects with the statin/fibrate combination are rare, but increased safety monitoring is advisable and the patient is warned to stop the drugs in the event of severe muscle pains and tenderness (Sampson & Betteridge 1999).

Although statins are among the best tolerated of all medicines, there are occasional patients who cannot tolerate them at all or who can tolerate only a small dose, insufficient to achieve the LDL goal. In these patients the cholesterol-lowering low-fat spreads containing stanol ester or sitosterols can be very helpful (Plat *et al.* 2000). These spreads lower the absorption of cholesterol and can reduce plasma LDL-cholesterol by 10–15 per cent if appropriate amounts are ingested. This reduction is equivalent to two dose doublings of statins. If further LDL-cholesterol lowering is required, the anion-exchange resins cholestyramine and colestipol are useful, if tolerated. They have the potential to interfere with the absorption of other drugs and need to be taken at least one hour before or four hours after concurrent medicines. For the patient completely intolerant of statins, the resins can be useful and can be combined with newer fibrates such as fenofibrate which are more effective at lowering LDL. For a detailed recent review of lipid-lowering drugs and dietary therapy, the reader is referred to an excellent article by Knopp (1999).

The treatment gap

The audit of risk factor management, ASPIRE (Aspire Steering Group 1996), highlighted the under-treatment of CHD patients with only a minority on statin drugs. Indeed, six months after major CHD events, 78 per cent of men and 86 per cent of women had a cholesterol reading of ≥ 5.5 mmol/l. One way of ensuring that CHD patients receive appropriate therapy is to start statins before hospital discharge. The joint British guidelines suggest that patients with a random total cholesterol concentration > 6.0 mmol/l should, in addition to dietary advice, receive a statin before discharge. At review (6–12 weeks post-discharge) those patients with cholesterol levels ≥ 5 mmol/l should also receive statins. The guidelines emphasise the opportunities for family screening of selected CHD patients to identify familial dyslipidaemias so that appropriate primary prevention may be instigated.

It is not just the UK that is failing to achieve optimal lipid-lowering therapy in secondary prevention. This is clear from the EuroAspire study which also showed under-treatment (EuroAspire Study Group 1997). Furthermore, a survey from the USA showed that only 16 per cent of high-risk patients were achieving LDL-cholesterol goals (Pearson *et al.* 2000). More recent data from the UK show only limited improvement in treatment rates (Primatesta & Poulter 2000).

Filling the treatment gap remains an important challenge for both primary and secondary care as outlined in the National Service Framework (Department of Health 2000). Discharging patients from coronary care units on statins is an important first step. Subsequent follow-up in primary care should ensure that adequate dosage is prescribed to achieve LDL targets. It is clear from market research data that the majority of patients still receive suboptimal doses.

Future directions

Ongoing trials will provide further important information which should influence clinical practice. Trials such as Treat to New Targets (TNT), Incremental Decrease in Endpoints Through Aggressive Lipid Lowering (IDEAL) and Study of the Effectiveness of Additional Reductions of Cholesterol and Homocysteine (SEARCH) address the question of how low to lower LDL-cholesterol in secondary prevention. There is a suggestion from the Post Coronary Artery Bypass Graft Trial Investigators (1997) that lower is better. In this angiographic trial more aggressive LDL lowering (target 2.4 mmol/l versus 3.4 mmol/l) was associated with a lower percentage of grafts showing progression of atherosclerosis, together with a reduction in revascularisation rates. The Atorvastatin Versus Revascularisation Treatment (AVERT) study provides further evidence that lower is better (Pitt *et al.* 1999). The trials in progress with large numbers of patients will provide definitive answers on this issue based on hard endpoints.

A large trial due to report in the autumn of 2001, the Heart Protection Study (HPS), should provide further information on the effects of cholesterol lowering (simvastatin 40 mg versus placebo) in a wide range of patients at high risk, including not only patients with established CHD but also those with occlusive disease of non-coronary arteries (MRC/BHF Heart Protection Collaborative Group 1999). Baseline cholesterol concentrations extend down to 3.5 mmol/l. This important study contains large numbers of patients with diabetes, together with large numbers of women and elderly people. More information in these groups will be welcome, particularly in women, given the disappointing outcome of the first hormone replacement therapy trial for secondary prevention (Hulley *et al.* 1998). HPS will also provide outcome data on an antioxidant cocktail containing vitamins E and C and β-carotene. The Prospective Study of Pravastatin in Elderly at Risk (PROSPER) has recruited a specifically elderly population (age range 70–82 years) and should provide important cost–benefit data on the treatment of this increasingly important population.

Conclusions

The case for lipid lowering and particularly LDL-cholesterol lowering in the secondary prevention of CHD is overwhelming (Pedersen 1998). Sadly there remains a huge treatment gap in the application of the findings of clinical science for the benefit of individual patients. Ongoing trials will provide further information on how aggressive LDL lowering should be for an important subgroup of the population. There is no doubt that the statins have transformed the treatment of CHD patients. That is not to say that nutritional and lifestyle measures are not important alongside drug therapy, but the recently announced preliminary results of MIRACL (Myocardial Ischaemia Reduction with Aggressive Cholesterol Lowering) at the American Heart Association meeting in New Orleans, November 2000, provide further testimony to the benefits of statins. In this trial high-dose statin (atorvastatin 80 mg versus placebo) was given immediately in acute coronary syndromes (non-Q wave myocardial infarction and unstable angina pectoris) and clinical endpoints were significantly reduced in as short a time as 16 weeks.

References

Aspire Steering Group (1996). A British Cardiac Society survey of the potential for the secondary prevention of coronary disease: ASPIRE (Action on secondary prevention through intervention to reduce events). Principal results. *Heart* **75**, 334–342

Assmann G, Schulte H, von Eckardstein A, Huang Y (1996). High density lipoprotein cholesterol as a predictor of coronary heart disease risk. The PROCAM experience and pathophysiological implications for reverse cholesterol transport. *Atherosclerosis* **124**(suppl), S11–S20

Bezafibrate Infarction Prevention (BIP) Study Group (2000). Secondary prevention by raising HDL cholesterol and reducing triglycerides in patients with coronary artery disease. *Circulation* **102**, 21–27

Brown G, Zhao Z-Q, Sacco DJ, Albers JJ (1993). Lipid lowering and plaque regression: new insights into prevention of plaque disruption and clinical events in coronary disease. *Circulation* **87**, 1781–1791

Department of Health (2000). *National Service Framework for Coronary Heart Disease.* London: HMSO

EuroAspire Study Group (1997). A European Society of Cardiology survey on secondary prevention of coronary heart disease: principal results. *European Heart Journal* **18**, 1569–1582

Durrington PN (1998). Triglycerides are more important in atherosclerosis than epidemiology has suggested. *Atherosclerosis* **141**(suppl), S57–S62

Goldberg RB, Mellies MJ, Sacks FM *et al.* (1998). Cardiovascular events and their reduction with pravastatin in diabetic and glucose-intolerant myocardial infarction survivors with average cholesterol levels: subgroup analyses in the Cholesterol and Recurrent Events (CARE) trial. *Circulation* **98**, 2513–2519

Haffner SM (2000). Secondary prevention of coronary heart disease. The role of fibric acids. *Circulation* **102**, 2–4

Haffner SM, Alexander CM, Cook TJ *et al.* (1999). Reduced coronary events in sim vastatin-treated patients with coronary heart disease and diabetes or impaired fasting glucose levels. Subgroup analyses in the Scandinavian Simvastatin Survival Study. *Archives of Internal Medicine* **159**, 2661–2667

Hokanson JE, Austin MA (1996). Plasma triglyceride level is a risk factor for cardiovascular disease independent of high density lipoprotein cholesterol level: a meta-analysis of population-based prospective studies. *Journal of Cardiovascular Risk* **3**, 213–219

Hulley SB, Roseman RH, Bawol RD, Brand RJ (1980). Epidemiology as a guide to clinical decisions. The association between triglyceride and coronary heart disease. *New England Journal of Medicine* **302**, 1383–1389

Hulley S, Grady D, Bush T *et al.* (1998). Randomized trial of oestrogen plus progestin for secondary prevention of coronary heart disease in postmenopausal women. *Journal of the American Medical Association* **280**, 605–613

Knopp RH (1999). Drug treatment of lipid disorders. *New England Journal of Medicine* **341**, 498–511

Kobashigawa JA, Katznelson S, Laks H *et al.* (1995). Effect of pravastatin on outcomes after cardiac transplantation. *New England Journal of Medicine* **333**, 621–627

Law M (2000). Lowering cardiovascular risk by cholesterol reduction: evidence from observational studies and randomised trials. In Betteridge DJ, ed., *Lipids and Vascular Disease: Current Issues*. London: Martin Dunitz, pp 173–182

Long-term Intervention with Pravastatin in Ischaemic Disease (LIPID) Study Group (1998). Prevention of cardiovascular events and death with pravastatin in patients with coronary heart disease and a broad range of initial cholesterol levels. *New England Journal of Medicine* **339**, 1349–1357

Miettinen TA, Pyörälä K, Olsson AG *et al.* (1997). Cholesterol-lowering therapy in women and elderly patients with myocardial infarction or angina pectoris. Scandinavian Simvastatin Survival Study (4S). *Circulation* **96**, 4211–4218

MRC/BHF Heart Protection Study Collaborative Group (1999). MRC/BHF Heart Protection Study of cholesterol-lowering therapy and of antioxidant vitamin supplementation in a wide range of patients at increased risk of coronary heart disease death: early safety and efficacy experience. *European Heart Journal* **20**, 725–741

Pearson TA, Laurora I, Chu H, Kafonek S (2000). The Lipid Treatment Assessment Project (L-TAP). A multicenter survey to evaluate the percentages of dyslipidemic patients receiving lipid-lowering therapy and achieving low-density lipoprotein cholesterol goals. *Archives of Internal Medicine* **160**, 459–467

Pedersen TR (1998). Aggressive lipid-lowering therapy: a clinical imperative. *European Heart Journal* **19**, M15–M21

Pekkanen J, Linn S, Heiss G *et al.* (1990). Ten year mortality from cardiovascular disease in relation to cholesterol level among men with and without pre existing cardiovascular disease. *New England Journal of Medicine* **322**, 1700–1701

Pitt B, Waters D, Brown WV *et al.* (1999). Aggressive lipid-lowering therapy compared with angioplasty in stable coronary artery disease. *New England Journal of Medicine* **342**, 70–76

Plat J, Kerckhoffs DAJM, Mensink RP (2000). Therapeutic potential of plant sterols and stanols. *Current Opinion in Lipidology* **11**, 571–576

Post Coronary Artery Bypass Graft Trial Investigators (1997). The effect of aggressive lowering of low density lipoprotein cholesterol levels and low dose anticoagulation on obstructive changes in saphenous vein coronary artery bypass grafts. *New England Journal of Medicine* **336**, 153–162

Primatesta P & Poulter NR (2000). Lipid concentrations and the use of lipid-lowering drugs: Evidence of a national cross-sectional survey. *British Medical Journal* **321**, 1322–1325

Pyörälä K, Pedersen TR, Kjekshus J, Faergman O, Olsson AG, Thorgeirsson G (1997). Cholesterol lowering with simvastatin improves rognosis of diabetic patients with coronary heart disease: a subgroup analysis of the Scandinavian Simvastatin Survival Study (4S). *Diabetes Care* **20**, 614–620

Ross R (1999). Atherosclerosis – an inflammatory disease. *New England Journal of Medicine* **340**, 115–126

Rossouw JE, Lewis B, Rifkind BM (1990) The value of lowering cholesterol after myocardial infarction. *New England Journal of Medicine* **323**, 1112–1119

Rubins HB, Robins SJ, Collins D *et al.* (1999). Gemfibrozil for the secondary prevention of coronary heart disease in men with low levels of high density lipoprotein cholesterol. *New England Journal of Medicine* **341**, 410–418

Sacks FM, Pfeffer MA, Moye LA *et al.* for the Cholesterol and Recurrent Events Trial Investigators (1996). The effect of pravastatin on coronary events after myocardial infarction in patients with average cholesterol levels. *New England Journal of Medicine* **335**, 1001–1009

Sampson MJ, Betteridge DJ (1999). Hyperlipidaemia and combination drug therapy. In Betteridge DJ, Illingworth DR, Shepherd J, eds, *Lipoproteins in Health and Disease.* London: Arnold, pp 1213–1229

Scandinavian Simvastatin Survival Study Group (1994). Randomised trial of cholesterol lowering in 4444 patients with coronary heart disease: the Scandinavian Simvastatin Survival Study (4S). *The Lancet* **344**, 1383–1389

Scandinavian Simvastatin Survival Study Group (1995). Baseline serum cholesterol and treatment effect in the Scandinavian Simvastatin Survival Study (4S). *The Lancet* **345**, 1274–1275

Superko HR, Krauss RM (1994). Coronary artery disease regression. Convincing evidence for the benefit of aggressive lipoprotein management. *Circulation* **90**, 1056–1069

Thompson GR (1997). What targets should lipid-modulating therapy achieve to optimise the prevention of coronary heart disease? *Atherosclerosis* **131**, 1–5

Wenke K, Meiser B, Thurg J *et al.* (1997). Simvastatin reduces graft vessel disease and mortality after heart transplantation: a four year randomized trial. *Circulation* **96**, 1398–1402

White HD, Simes RJ, Anderson NE *et al.* (2000). Pravastatin therapy and the risk of stroke. *New England Journal of Medicine* **343**, 317–326

Wood D, Durrington P, Poulter N, McInnes G, Rees A, Wray R (1998). Joint British recommendations on prevention of coronary heart disease in clinical practice. *Heart* **80**(suppl 2), S1–S29

Chapter 4

Effective secondary prevention: the place of aspirin, ACE inhibition and β blockade

Carol Fisher and John JV McMurray

Introduction

Despite falling population mortality rates from coronary heart disease, myocardial infarction remains common and deadly. At least 25 per cent of patients die rapidly, before hospital admission is possible (Macintyre *et al.* 2001). As around two-thirds of patients having a myocardial infarction (MI) have already been identified as having coronary heart disease (CHD) (Tunstall Pedoe *et al.* 1975), many of these out-of-hospital deaths are avoidable. Of patients admitted to hospital, 25 per cent die within 30 days. Of those discharged alive from hospital, 31.4 per cent die within one year and 64 per cent by ten years (Capewell *et al.* 2000). There is, therefore, enormous scope for further improving prognosis through acute treatments and long-term secondary prevention after MI. Sadly, recent data suggest that many patients in the UK are still denied these life-saving measures (EUROASPIRE 2001). This chapter summarises the evidence that antiplatelet therapy, β blockers and angiotensin-converting enzyme (ACE) inhibitors improve prognosis after MI.

Antiplatelet therapy

Aspirin

Although early administration of aspirin as a treatment for acute MI reduces immediate (ISIS-2 Collaborative Group 1988) and longer-term (ten-year) mortality (ISIS-2 Collaborative Group 1998) (despite only being administered for five weeks), there is less evidence that chronic administration of aspirin after five weeks is of prognostic benefit. Current recommendations to prescribe long-term aspirin therapy to MI survivors are based on the Anti-platelet Trialists' Collaboration (ATC 1994) meta-analysis. This examined 145 randomised trials of antiplatelet therapy versus controls. These trials included 70,000 high-risk patients, i.e. patients known to have vascular disease or other conditions that imply an increased risk of occlusive vascular disease. Of about 20,000 patients with acute MI, 10 per cent of patients on antiplatelet therapy suffered a vascular event compared with 14 per cent of patients in the control group, i.e. about 40 vascular events can be avoided per 1,000 patients treated ($2p < 0.00001$). Vascular events were defined as non-fatal MIs, non-fatal strokes or vascular deaths. Among 20,000 patients with a past history of MI, 13 per cent of patients receiving antiplatelet therapy suffered a vascular event compared with 17 per cent in the control group, i.e. a two-year benefit of about 40 vascular events avoided per 1,000 patients treated ($2p < 0.00001$) (Figure 4.1). Vascular events were therefore reduced by about a quarter and significantly so in all important subgroups of patients, e.g. middle age and older age, men and women, hypertensive and normotensive patients, and diabetic and non-diabetic patients.

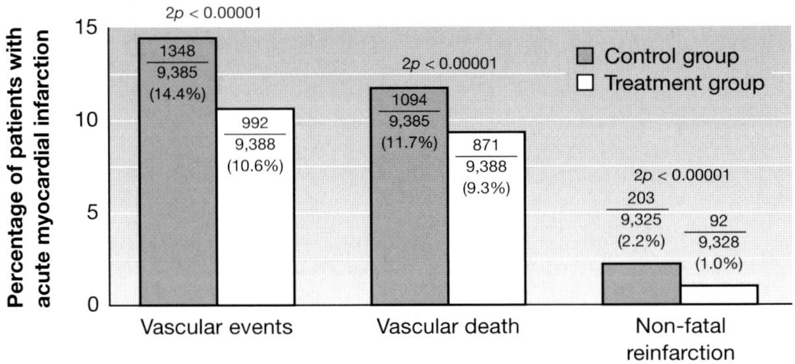

Figure 4.1 Reductions in vascular events (myocardial infarction, stroke, vascular death), vascular deaths and non-fatal reinfarctions in 18,773 patients with suspected acute myocardial infarction caused by prophylaxis with antiplatelet medication (mostly aspirin), compared with control (placebo or no antiplatelet medication). Average follow-up 2.4 years. (Adapted from Antiplatelet Trialists' collaboration 1994)

Clopidogrel

Clopidogrel is a thienopyridine derivative that inhibits platelet aggregation induced by adenosine diphosphate (Figure 4.2). The **C**lopidogrel **a**nd **P**revention of **R**ecurrent **I**schaemic **E**vents (CAPRIE) study (CAPRIE 1996) compared clopidogrel 75 mg with aspirin 325 mg (both taken once daily) in 19,185 patients with arterial disease (recent ischaemic stroke, recent MI or symptomatic peripheral arterial disease). The primary end-point was a composite of vascular death, MI or ischaemic stroke. After an average follow-up of 1.9 years, the annualised risk was 5.83 per cent in the aspirin group and 5.32 per cent in the clopidogrel group, a relative risk reduction of 8.7 per cent ($p = 0.043$) (Figure 4.3). Not surprisingly, given its mode of action and the dose used, aspirin caused more gastric side effects. The evidence that clopidogrel is an efficacious antiplatelet agent has recently been reinforced by the Clopidogrel in Unstable Angina to Prevent Recurrent Events study (CURE 2001).

In this study clopidogrel *added* to aspirin significantly reduced major vascular events in patients with acute coronary syndromes (non-ST segment elevation MI and unstable angina). A loading dose of 300 mg followed by 75 mg clopidogrel daily was given. The dose of aspirin given was 75–325 mg daily alone or in combination. Average follow-up was nine months. A 20 per cent relative risk reduction in

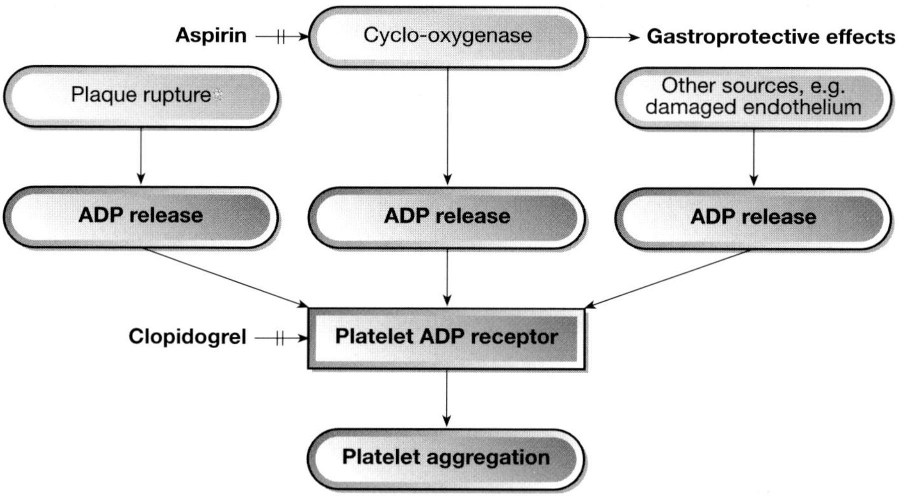

Figure 4.2 Mode of action of aspirin and clopidogrel. SAVE = Survival and Ventricular Enlargement; AIRE = Acute Infarction Ramipril Efficacy; TRACE = trandolapril in patients with reduced left-ventricular function after acute myocardial infarction

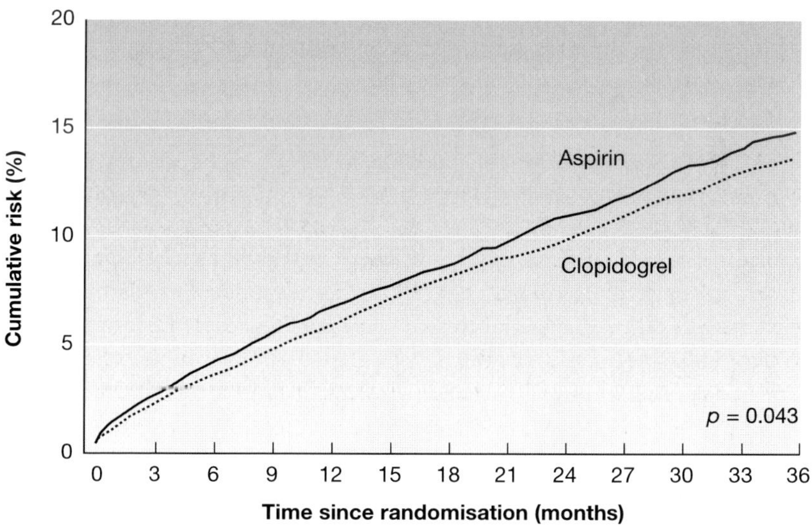

Figure 4.3 Cumulative risk of ischaemic stroke, myocardial infarction or vascular death. (Adapted from the CAPRIE Study 1996)

cardiovascular death, MI or stroke was found in the combination group (9.3% in the combination group versus 11.5% in the aspirin group). However, a 30 per cent increase in bleeding was found in the combination group. Treating 1,000 patients for nine months would therefore prevent 28 major events in 23 patients at a cost of three life-threatening bleeds and three other transfusions.

Consequently, clopidogrel is a more expensive alternative to aspirin in aspirin-intolerant patients. The place of clopidogrel as an antiplatelet agent to use in addition to aspirin in the long term has yet to be determined.

Recommendations

All patients should receive life-long aspirin therapy or clopidogrel if aspirin intolerant.

ACE inhibitors

Three large trials (GISSI-3 1994; ISIS-4 1995; CCS-1 1997) have shown that short-term, early use of ACE inhibitors over the first few days and weeks after acute MI leads to a small but significant reduction in mortality (similar to that seen with intravenous β blockers), a conclusion supported by a recent meta-analysis (ACE Inhibitor Myocardial Infarction Collaborative Group 1998).

Three large trials have also shown that ACE inhibitor therapy, started in the first few days and weeks and continued long term, substantially reduces morbidity and mortality in *high-risk* MI survivors (Figure 4.4). These trials identified high-risk patients on the basis of having left ventricular systolic dysfunction (LVSD) or evidence of acute heart failure (AHF) complicating MI. These studies and others have been included in a recent meta-analysis (Flather *et al.* 2000). Overall there was a 28 per cent reduction in death, MI and hospital admissions for heart failure in

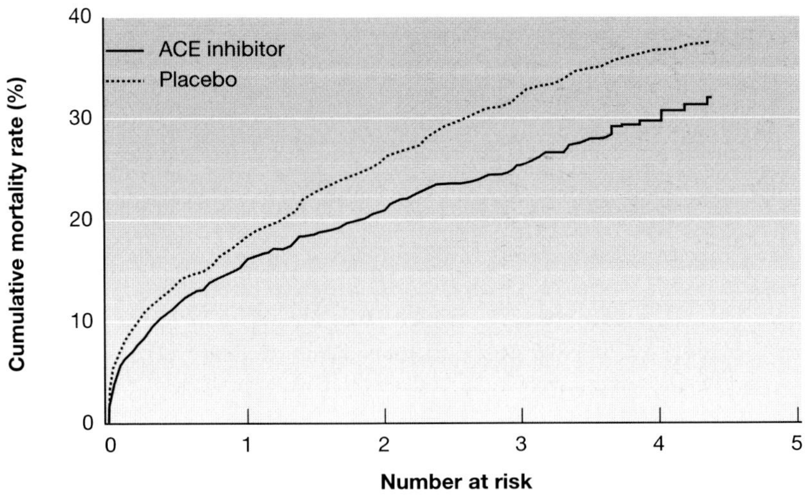

Figure 4.4 Adapted from systematic overview of ACE inhibitor therapy

patients with LVSD after MI treated with ACE inhibitors. This equates 70 patients with at least one event prevented for every 1,000 patients treated. Consequently, all such high-risk MI survivors should receive life-long ACE inhibitor treatment.

We did not know, however, until recently, whether other MI survivors (i.e. those without LVSD or AHF) should receive life-long treatment with an ACE inhibitor. The Heart Outcomes Prevention Evaluation (HOPE) study (2000) has answered this question. In HOPE, 9,297 patients at high risk of vascular events (by virtue of having prior stroke/transient ischaemic attack [TIA], coronary heart disease [CHD], peripheral arterial disease or diabetes plus another vascular risk factor) were randomised to placebo or ramipril (target dose 10 mg once daily). The primary end-point was a composite of cardiovascular death, MI and stroke. After an average follow-up of five years, the cumulative event rate was 17.8 per cent in the placebo group and 14 per cent in the ramipril group ($p < 0.001$). All-cause mortality was also reduced (from 12.2% to 10.4%, $p = 0.005$) as was the need for 'revascularisation procedures', e.g. percutaneous coronary intervention, coronary artery bypass surgery (from 18.3% to 16%, $p = 0.002$) (Figure 4.5).

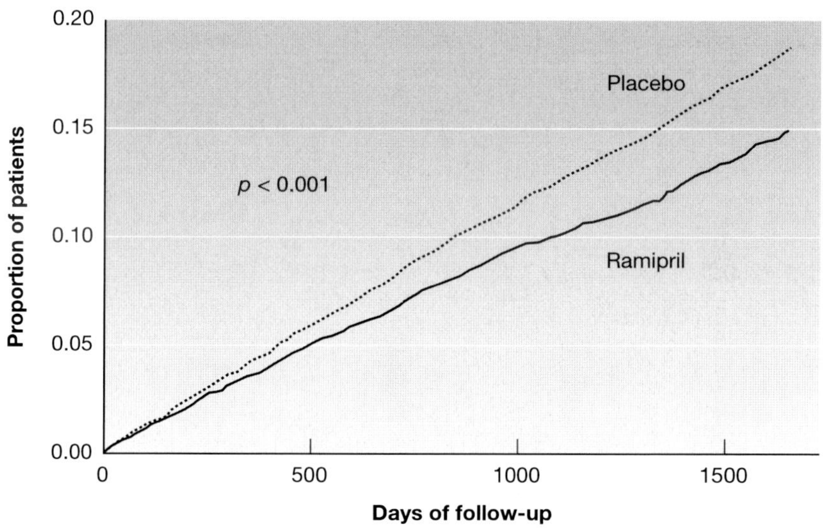

Figure 4.5 The HOPE study: Kaplan–Meier estimates of the composite outcome of myocardial infarction, stroke or death from cardiovascular causes in the ramipril group and the placebo group; $p < 0.001$. (Adapted from the HOPE study 2000)

Recommendations

Collectively, these striking and consistent treatment effects support the use of life-long ACE inhibitor treatment in all MI survivors.

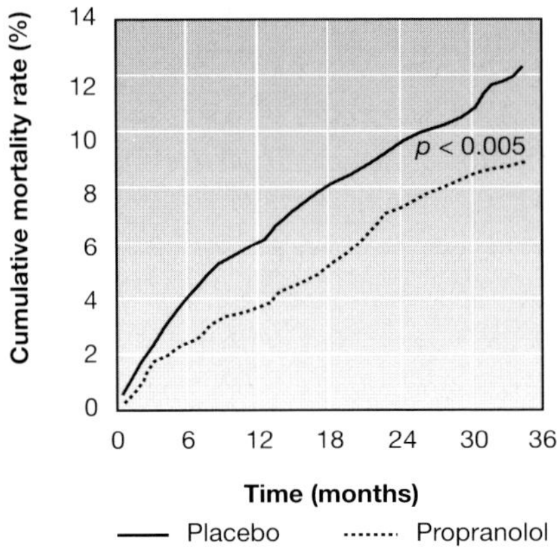

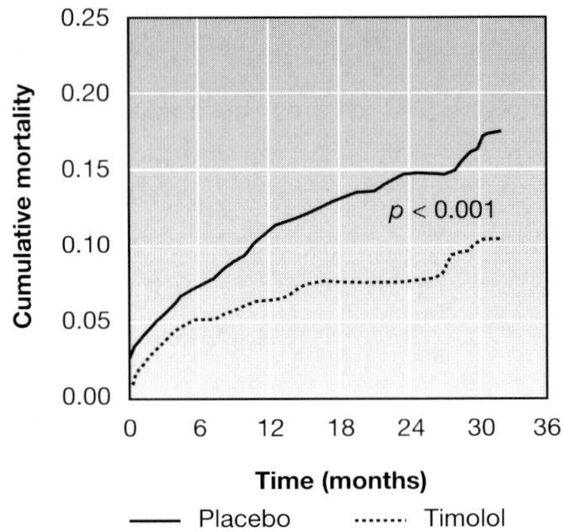

Figure 4.6 (a) Cumulative mortality after myocardial infarction in the Beta-blocker Heart Attack Trial (BHAT). (Adapted from BHAT Research Group 1982.)
(b) Norwegian Multi-Centre Timolol Study (1981)

β-Adrenoreceptor antagonists (β blockers)

The ISIS-1 study showed that treatment of patients with acute MI with early intravenous atenolol led to a small but significant reduction in mortality. Two landmark trials (Figure 4.6), the β Blocker Heart Attack Trial (with propranolol: BHAT 1982) and the Norwegian Multi Centre Timolol Study (1981), further showed that oral β-blocker therapy, started within a few days to weeks after MI, and continued long term, substantially and significantly reduced the risk of death and recurrent MI. Other trials and meta-analyses supported these findings (Freemantle *et al.* 1999).

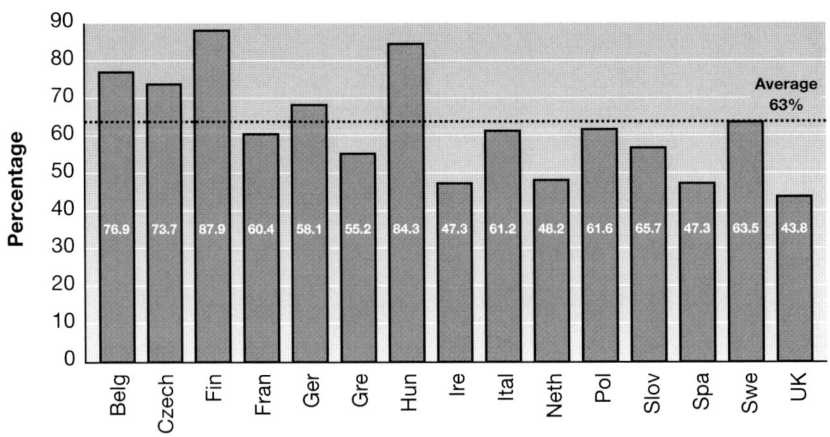

Figure 4.7 EUROASPIRE II: β blocker use at interview

β Blockers are not, however, as widely used post-MI as they should be, especially in the UK (Figure 4.7). Why this is so is unclear. Some have taken the view that such 'old' studies are no longer relevant in the modern era of MI management (these older studies were conducted at a time when aspirin, thrombolysis, ACE inhibitors and statins were not used).

In the light of this the Carvedilol Post Infarct Survival Control In Left Ventricular Dysfunction study (CAPRICORN 2001) was recently undertaken. This study focused on high-risk post-MI patients with significant LVSD. These higher-risk patients, many of whom also develop acute heart failure, were probably excluded from the earlier β-blocker trials. Recent trials have shown that ACE inhibitors substantially reduce morbidity and mortality in these patients (see above).

Consequently, CAPRICORN randomised patients with acute MI, complicated by LVSD, to either placebo (n = 984) or carvedilol (n = 975), given in *addition* to full conventional therapy, including an ACE inhibitor. After an average follow-up of 1.3 years, 116 (12%) patients in the carvedilol group and 151 (15%) in the placebo group died, i.e. mortality was reduced by 23 per cent (p = 0.03). Non-fatal reinfarction occurred in 34 (3%) in the carvedilol group and 57 (6%) in the placebo group, i.e. 41 per cent reduction (p = 0.014) (Figure 4.8).

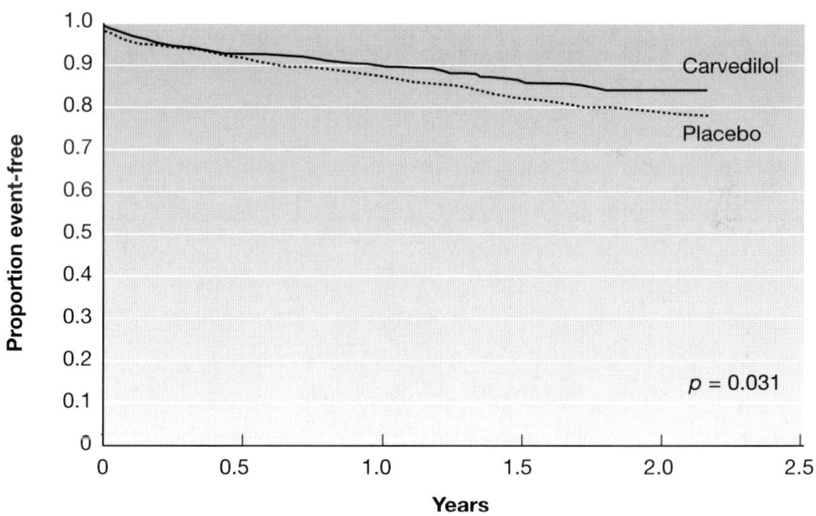

Figure 4.8 CAPRICORN Study: Kaplan–Meier estimates of all-cause mortality. (Adapted from CAPRICORN Study 2001)

This important new trial reiterates the value of β blockers post-MI, even in the modern era of MI management (Figure 4.9).

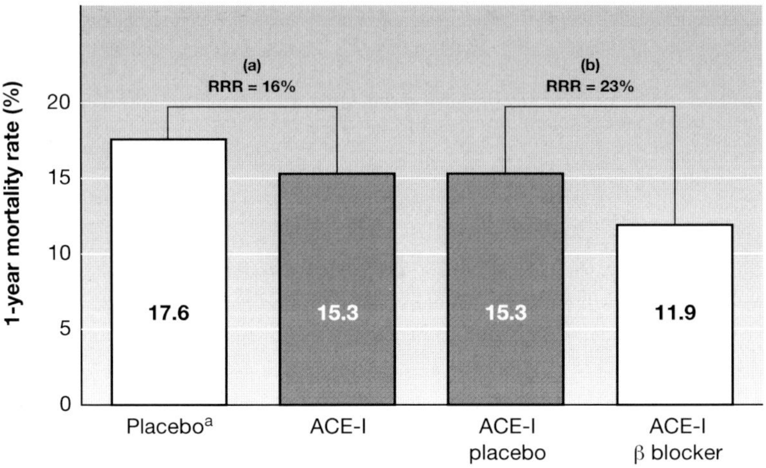

Figure 4.9 Potential incremental mortality reductions with ACE inhibition and β-blocker therapy in high-risk survivors of myocardial infarction. (a) SAVE/AIRE/TRACE 1992–95; (b) CAPRICORN 2001. [a]Twenty-five per cent on β blocker. RRR = relative risk reduction. SAVE, Survival and Ventricular Enlargement; AIRE, Acute Infarction Ramipril Efficacy; TRACE, trandolapril in patients with reduced left-ventricular function after acute myocardial infarction

Recommendations

There is now overwhelming evidence that virtually all patients should receive life-long treatment with a β blocker post-MI.

The only absolute contraindication to β-blocker therapy is asthma.

Summary and conclusions

Around half of the recent reduction in coronary heart disease mortality in the UK and elsewhere has resulted from acute treatments for MI and secondary prevention measures (Capewell & McMurray 1999; Capewell *et al.* 2000). The individual and cumulative mortality and morbidity reductions with secondary prevention treatments are substantial (Table 4.1) (McMurray 1998).

There is still widespread underuse of secondary prevention measures and their increased use could lead to further large benefits (Capewell *et al.* 1999). There is an overwhelming evidence base for β-blocker and ACE inhibitor therapy post-MI and a somewhat less substantial one for antiplatelet therapy. These and other measures must be systematically employed post-MI, as recommended in UK national guidelines (Table 4.2) (NSF CHD 2000; SIGN 2000; NICE 2001). Already, in Scotland, the process of a national audit of the effectiveness of hospitals in implementing

Table 4.1 Benefits of evidence-based secondary prevention

Treatment	*Problems prevented per 1,000 patient-years of treatment*
Oral β blockers (low-risk patients)	13 deaths/5 MI
Oral β blockers (high-risk patients)	27 deaths/18 MI
Aspirin	16 deaths/MI/strokes
HMG-CoA reductase inhibitor	6 deaths/12 MI/4 CHF/11 revascularisations[a]
Smoking cessation	27 deaths
ACE inhibitor – low LVEF (SAVE)	12 deaths/9 MI/ 16 CHF/10 revascularisations[a]
ACE inhibitor – low WMI (TRACE)	46 deaths/24 CHF
ACE inhibitor – heart failure (AIRE)	45 deaths/26 CHF

ACE, angiotensin-converting enzyme; CHF, chronic heart failure;
HMG-CoA, hydroxymethylglutaryl-coenzyme A; LVEF, left ventricular ejection fraction;
MI, myocardial infarction; WMI, wall motion index.
[a]Revascularisation = coronary angioplasty or bypass surgery.

Table 4.2 Comparison of national guidelines for pharmacological intervention following myocardial infarction

	Aspirin should be considered in	*β Blocker should be considered in*	*ACE inhibitor should be considered in*
SIGN	All patients	All patients	All patients
NICE	All patients	All patients	All patients
NSF	All patients	All patients	Patients with evidence of LVSD

ACE, angiotensin-converting enzyme; LVSD, left ventricular systolic dysfunction;
NICE, National Institute for Clinical Excellence; NSF, National Service Framework;
SIGN, Scottish Intercollegiate Guidelines Network.

secondary preventive measures post-MI has been completed by the Clinical Standards Board (2000). A public report of hospital performance will be published by the end of 2001. Similar implementation schemes will be enacted in other parts of the UK.

References

ACE Inhibitor Myocardial Infarction Collaborative Group (1998). Indications for ACE inhibitors in the Early Treatment of Acute Myocardial Infarction. *Circulation* **97**, 2202–2212

Antiplatelet Trialists' Collaboration (1994). Collaborative overview of randomised trials of antiplatelet therapy. Prevention of death, myocardial infarction and stroke by prolonged antiplatelet therapy in various categories of patients. *British Medical Journal* **308**, 81–106

BHAT Research Group (1982). A randomised trial of propranolol in patients with acute myocardial infarction. *Journal of the American Medical Association* **247**, 1707–1714

Capewell S & McMurray JJV (1999). Contribution of modern cardiovascular treatment and risk factor changes to the decline in CHD mortality in Scotland 1975–1994. *Heart* **81**, 380–386

Capewell S, Pell J, Morrison C, McMurray J (1999). Increasing the impact of cardiological treatments. How best to reduce deaths. *European Heart Journal* **20**, 1386–1392

Capewell S, Livingston BM, MacIntyre K *et al.* (2000). Trends in case fatality in 117,718 patients admitted with acute myocardial infarction in Scotland. *European Heart Journal* **21**, 1833–1840

CAPRICORN Investigators (2001). Effect of Carvedilol on outcome after myocardial infarction in patients with left-ventricular dysfunction: the CAPRICORN randomised trial. *The Lancet* **357**, 1385–1390

CAPRIE Steering Committee (1996). Clopidogrel versus aspirin in patients at risk of ischaemic events. *The Lancet* **348**, 1329–1339

Chinese Cardiac Study 1 (CCS-1) (1997). Oral captopril versus placebo among 14,962 patients with suspected acute myocardial infarction: a multicenter, randomised, double-blind, placebo controlled clinical trial. Chinese Cardiac Study (CCS-1) Collaborative Group. *Chinese Medical Journal* (English) **110**, 834–838

Clinical Standards Board for Scotland (2000). *Secondary Prevention Following Acute Myocardial Infarction*. Edinburgh. December. www.clinicalstandards.org

CURE Study (2001). Effects of clopidogrel in addition to aspirin in patients with acute coronary syndromes without ST-segment elevation. The Clopidogrel in Unstable Angina to Prevent Recurrent Ischaemic Events Trial Investigators. *New England Journal of Medicine* **345**, 494–502

EUROASPIRE (2001). Lifestyle and risk factor management and use of drug therapies in coronary patients from 15 countries: principal results from EUROASPIRE II (European Heart Survey Programme). *European Heart Journal* **22**, 554–572

Flather M, Yusuf S, Kober L, Pfeffer M *et al.* (2000). Long-term ACE-inhibitor therapy in patients with heart failure or left-ventricular dysfunction: a systematic overview of data from individual patients. *The Lancet* **355**, 1575–1581

Freemantle N, Cleland J, Young P, Mason J, Harrison J (1999). Beta blockade after myocardial infarction: systemic review and meta regression analysis. *British Medical Journal* **318**, 1730–1737

Gruppo Italiano per lo Studio della Sopravvivenza nell'Infarcto miocardico (GISSI-3) Study Group (1994). Effects of lisinopril and transdermal glyceryl trinitrate singly and together on 6 week mortality and ventricular function after myocardial infarction. *The Lancet* **343**, 1115–1122

Heart Outcomes Prevention Evaluation Study Investigators (2000). Effects of an angiotensin-converting-enzyme inhibitor, ramipril, on cardiovascular events in high risk patients. *New England Journal of Medicine* **342**, 145–153

ISIS-2 Collaborative Group (1988). Randomised trial of streptokinase, oral aspirin, both or neither among 17,187 cases of suspected acute myocardial infarction. *The Lancet* **ii**, 349–360.

ISIS-2 Collaborative Group (1998). Ten year survival among patients with suspected myocardial infarction in randomised comparison of intravenous streptokinase, oral aspirin or neither. The ISIS-2 (Second International Study of Infarct Survival) Collaborative Group. *British Medical Journal* **316**, 1337–1343

ISIS-4 Collaborative Group (1995). A randomised factorial trial assessing early oral captopril, oral mononitrate and intravenous magnesium sulphate in 58,050 patients with suspected acute myocardial infarction. *The Lancet* **345**, 669–685

MacIntyre K, Stewart S, Chalmers J *et al.* (2001). Relationship between socioeconomic deprivation and death from a first myocardial infarction in Scotland: population based analysis. *British Medical Journal* **322**, 1152–1153

McMurray JJV (1998). *Secondary Prevention Post MI.* London: Martin Dunitz

National Institute for Clinical Excellence (2001). *Prophylaxis for Patients Who Have Experienced a Myocardial Infarction: Drug treatment, cardiac rehabilitation and dietary manipulation.* NICE, London, April. www.nice.org.uk

National Service Framework for Coronary Heart Disease (2000). Department of Health, London. March www.doh.gov.uk/nsf/coronary.htm

Norwegian Multi Centre Timolol Study (1981). *New England Journal of Medicine* **309**, 801–807

Scottish Intercollegiate Guidelines Network (2000). *Secondary Prevention of Coronary Heart Disease. Following myocardial infarction.* SIGN, Edinburgh. January www.sign.ac.uk

Tunstall Pedoe H, Clayton D, Morris J, Brigden W, McDonald L (1975). Coronary heart attacks in East London. *The Lancet* **i**, 833

PART 4

Evidence and opinion for surgical intervention

Chapter 5

Evidence for effectiveness of coronary artery surgery in secondary prevention

Tom Treasure

Introduction

Coronary artery surgery is highly effective in relieving the symptom of angina and thus 'preventing' its re-occurrence. There is ample evidence that surgical relief of angina results in a much improved quality of life (Pocock *et al.* 1996). Furthermore, the benefits are related to the adequacy of revascularisation and are lost when vein grafts become diseased and occlude. The operation is dramatically effective in delivering a mechanistic solution to a mechanical problem, i.e. restoring blood flow to the ischaemic myocardium.

Coronary artery surgery also has an established role in reducing the risk of death. Put simply, patients who have features that distinguish them as having a predictably high incidence of future life-threatening events can be made safer by surgery.

However, by 'secondary prevention' we mean a strategy that can be applied across the board to reduce coronary events and thus avert death and myocardial infarction. In this role the author argues that coronary artery surgery is largely ineffective.

Ideal secondary prevention would have no risk, and no cost implications. Altering diet for coronary surgery almost certainly fulfils both of these criteria. Aspirin is low cost and low risk. In the scheme of things, major surgery must be regarded as high risk and high cost.

Surgery as secondary prevention?

To understand the issues, a distinction has to be drawn between surgery for symptoms and surgery for survival. A good example of major surgery for symptoms is hip replacement. In these, patients' survival is almost completely independent of the osteoarthritis of their hip joints. There is a small operative mortality and some unoperated patients might conceivably perish from pulmonary embolism as a consequence of immobility, but the considerations are almost exclusively the severity of pain and mobility. These symptoms are predictably relieved by hip replacement. The impact of an osteoarthritic hip on survival is not a factor in the decision to provide surgery for an individual or a population.

There are other operations performed purely or predominantly for prognosis. Carotid artery surgery is a useful example, and has been the subject of multicentre trials in Europe and North America (Easton & Wilterdink 1994). The operation is done to prevent stroke. It is a high-cost and high-risk procedure. Used indiscriminately in patients with an inherently low risk of stroke, it would cause more strokes than it prevents. Even in patients with significant carotid stenoses, many carotid endarterectomies must be performed for each stroke prevented, in some categories as many as 80 operations to prevent a single stroke.

The 'saving lives' argument for increasing the general provision of coronary artery surgery and reducing waiting lists is commonplace, emotionally compelling and seems to be generally accepted. The author argues that it is largely erroneous. Even those who agree that the shroud-waving argument is not sustainable on the evidence argue that an attention grabbing 'People Are Dying' banner headline is the only language that politicians understand. In order to provide more surgery for the relief of angina (which is fully justified) they argue for a maximisation of the impact of the fear of death. The author cannot share that view – if we are to be respected we must do it by compelling, logical and scientifically sound arguments. We should not use our powerful influence as doctors to push a false argument. Furthermore this approach has the inevitable consequence that it frightens rather than reassures many patients.

Three forms of evidence are presented:

- evidence from randomised trials;
- published waiting list mortality data;
- how this fits with an understanding of the inter-relationship of the pathology of coronary atherosclerosis, the symptom of angina and the likelihood of myocardial infarction.

Randomised trials of the effect of coronary artery surgery on survival

Coronary artery surgery flourished in the 1970s and mortality rates fell to very low levels. Many surgeons were able to publish series with mortality figures approaching zero. Practice at that time was selective. We were already well versed in the incremental risk factors for perioperative death and sought to avoid them. Those related to the patient's cardiac status were (and still are) an already damaged left ventricle, diffuse disease into the distal vessels and diabetes. Others that are now politically incorrect were age, and at the time elderly was over 65, and female sex. Both were excluded in the European trial. The boundaries of surgical indication were pushed in the direction of milder disease, and less angina, as the belief grew that this highly effective, very reproducible and impressively safe operation would also save lives by preventing future episodes of infarction.

This belief was put to the test by the North American Coronary Artery Surgery Study (CASS) in which patients with mild or moderate angina were randomised to either an initial strategy of surgical or of medical management. At five years, and at every point beyond that, there was absolutely no difference in survival between the two groups, irrespective of whether they had one-, two- or three-vessel disease. At five years only 25 of 258 patients with three-vessel disease had died, about 2 per cent per annum with deaths occurring at the same low rate whether they had been operated upon or not (CASS Principal Investigators *et al.* 1984)

It seemed to some inexplicable that these patients with significant coronary atherosclerosis, the biggest single killer in the developed world, appeared so remarkably safe, so safe that even a low-risk operation did not make them safer. Something must have gone wrong with the trial. To understand the paradox a number of very important facts must be taken into account. These were highly selected patients. The patients randomised into the trial were only 5 per cent of the cases included in the trial register. Patients with left main stem stenosis, many others whose doctors felt should have grafts and any patients with more than moderate angina were excluded from randomisation and were operated upon. This was in a way a trial of secondary prevention. It asked whether a strategem of surgery based simply on bypassing discovered coronary stenoses would save lives. The answer was that it did not.

Other trials were more inclusive. For example, the Veterans Administration trial included left main stem stenosis and the European study patients had much worse angina (Kumar & Treasure 1996). Yusuf *et al.* (1994) performed a meta-analysis of the 2,650 patients included in the three large and several other smaller trials and found that, by five years, the death rate in the medical group was 3.2 per cent overall compared with 2 per cent by an initial treatment strategy of immediate surgery. That means that on the basis of 'number needed to treat' 83 coronary operations must be performed to save one life a year. That is a very expensive strategy for secondary prevention.

Waiting list data

Apart from the banner headlines there is not much evidence that patients die on the waiting list. The waiting list is of course selected. Cardiologists, surgeons and indeed patients themselves have had to accept the view that the risk of death is not high. We have already selected out those in whom we believe life is in danger.

All 13 cardiac surgery centres in the Netherlands participated in an audit of deaths on the waiting list (Plomp *et al.* 1999). They discovered that, for patients on the waiting list for 12 weeks or more, the death rate was 0.68 per 1,000 patient weeks, a rate of about 3.5 per cent. This is remarkably similar to the death rate in the meta-analysis of patients who were randomised to the medical arm of the trials. It gives a degree of corroboration that the evidence in the trials can be generalised.

In the Dutch study the death rate was higher in the first two weeks of the waiting list. There were 80 deaths among 67,217 patients in their first month on the waiting list, including those selected for early surgery on the basis of recognised danger signals. The death rate in the first month was 1.2 per cent. It is hard to wave a convincing shroud about that when the present mortality rate for coronary surgery is 2–3 per cent in hospital or within 30 days of surgery.

New Zealand has addressed priority for coronary surgery on the basis of risk of waiting and the greater the degree of benefit in terms of angina relief and return to active life. During a median wait of 146 days there were 18 deaths with a risk per month of 0.28 per cent (Seddon *et al.* 1999). The actual waiting list mortality was 2.6–3.4 per cent per annum if the monthly risk is multiplied up. Again the figure is close to that in the trials. The number needed to treat to save a life a year is thus about 65 of these patients deemed safe enough to wait.

It is tragic for a patient and their family to be advised to have surgery and then to die before the day comes. However, patients also die having surgery. Furthermore there is a steady death rate after surgery at the rate of about 2 per cent per annum. The evidence from both trials and waiting list data is that a strategy of surgery aimed at secondary prevention is unlikely to be regarded as cost-effective. If surgery is the best management of angina for that individual, why suffer symptoms for a year or more waiting? But that is a different argument.

Atheroma, angina and coronary deaths

Why is there an idea that so many angina suffers are in imminent risk of death? An appealingly simple answer is to think about coronary artery disease as the linear cause and effect model:

- a lot of people have **atherosclerosis** of their coronary arteries;
- when this is bad enough they get **angina;**
- complete blocks cause **myocardial infarction;**
- these otherwise 'well' people then **die** of myocardial infarction.

The apparently self-evident conclusion is that death can be averted if the coronary arteries are bypassed before stage 3 is reached. The logic is that if, we intervene with revascularisation between steps 2 and 3, lives will be saved in large numbers. Indeed, our cardiological and surgical colleagues go to the press with monotonous regularity telling the world that patients are dying on waiting lists and those lives could be saved by intervention. The flaw is that, although each statement (1–4) is independently true, the sequence is broken more often than followed and nature is unpredictable at every step.

The problem is that states 1–4 do not follow each other in this orderly sequence. It does not go atherosclerosis → angina → myocardial infarction → death. Instead think of a Venn diagram constructed as follows:

1. Circle 1: a lot of people have **atherosclerosis** of their coronary arteries. Many die with atherosclerosis never having had angina or myocardial infarction. This is a big circle.

2. Circle 2: **angina** is a condition that may afflict the sufferer over a period of decades. In all but a few cases it affects people who have atherosclerosis of the coronary arteries. It is a smaller circle largely within but a small part outside C1. Angina may be episodic, i.e. some periods of life with and some periods without angina. For practical purposes we could define C2 as including all people who ever had angina.
3. Circle 3: **myocardial infarction** is an event that usually (but not always) afflicts people with atherosclerosis. C3 is therefore also largely within C1. It overlaps C2 because some have had angina but for many it is the first manifestation. An important fact to remember is that in cases where the coronary anatomy is known and who subsequently infarct, it as likely to be the mild stenosis (not causing angina) as the tight ('culprit') stenosis that causes infarct (Patterson & Treasure 1991).
4. Circle 4: these are people who **die** as a result of a coronary artery stenosis who therefore are candidates for saving by surgery (or for that matter angioplasty). They must all be within C1 because atherosclerosis is a requirement to receive the intervention (leaving aside very unusual reasons such as bridged or aberrant coronary arteries). Some will have had angina so it must overlap with C2. Some will have had an MI so it must overlap with C3. Some have had both so it overlaps the C2/C3 overlap. Many of those who die (C4) have had neither.

Whom should we target to save life?

Coronary artery disease is unpredictable. There is no reliable relationship among atherosclerosis, angina and death. Fatal coronary events, with plaque fissuring and thrombosis, may hit any plaque, whether it is haemodynamically insignificant or severe, whether it is in a relatively safe site (small branch to non-critical territory) or a life-threatening one (proximal left anterior descending or LAD), and at any time. We can treat angina by restoring flow to the ischaemic area but preventing death is less certain.

Absent from recent trials and scarce in older trials are the patients in whom we believe coronary revascularisation has a preventative role. The more severe subsets are not put on waiting lists.

The recognised patient descriptors are under three headings:

- dangerous coronary anatomy;
- low ischaemic threshold;
- an already damaged left ventricle.

Under each of these headings we can define criteria that alone or in combination make the likelihood of death sufficiently high that surgery should be considered to improve prognosis. However, trials have typically taken the safest and most stable patients, only 3–5 per cent of those eligible, so the patients most at risk and therefore with the most to gain, have often been excluded.

Randomised controlled trials have shown that surgery and angioplasty are similar in risk but that angioplasty fails much more often in keeping the treated coronary arteries open (Kumar & Treasure 1996). Any shortcomings in surgery will apply more so to PTCA as a secondary prevention.

Conclusion

As has been shown, published data on waiting list deaths show a rate of about 3.5 per cent per annum, uncannily close to the repeatedly observed background death rate in the medical and postoperative limbs of randomised trials. The background death rate for patients with the mildest coronary disease, or who have been successfully revascularised, is approximately 2 per cent. The margin of benefit is so small that it would take about 65 operations to save a life in these patients.

It should not be forgotten that there are well-defined groups of patients who should be offered surgery because they face an annual death rate of nearer 10 per cent and very many more for whom surgery offers excellent relief of symptoms. It is already proven that surgery cannot improve on that mortality rate.

References

CASS Principal Investigators *et al.* (1984). Myocardial infarction and mortality in the Coronary Artery Surgery Study (CASS) Randomized Trial. *New England Journal of Medicine* **310**, 750–758

Easton JD & Wilterdink JL (1994). Carotid endarterectomy: Trials and tribulations. *Annals of Neurology* **35**, 5–17

Kumar P & Treasure T (1996). Coronary artery bypass graft trials. *British Journal of Heart Medicine* **56**, 33–36

Patterson DL & Treasure T (1991). The culprit coronery artery lesion. *The Lancet* **338**, 1379–1380

Plomb J, Redekop WK, Dekker FW *et al.* (1991). Death on the waiting list for cardiac surgery in The Netherlands in 1994 and 1995. *Heart* **8**, 593–597

Pocock SJ, Henderson RA, Seed P, Treasure T, Hampton JR (1996). Quality of life, employment status and anginal symptoms after coronary angioplasty or bypass surgery: three years follow-up in the Randomised Intervention Treatment of Angina (RITA) Trial. *Circulation* **94**, 135–142

Seddon ME, French JK, Amos DJ, Ramanathan K, McLaughlin SC, White HD (1999). Waiting times and priorization for coronary artery bypass surgery in New Zealand. *Heart* **81**, 586–592

Yusuf S, Zucker D, Peduzzi P *et al.* (1994). Effect of coronary artery bypass graft surgery on survival: overview of 10-year results from randomized trials by the Coronary Artery Bypass Graft Surgery Trialists Collaboration. *The Lancet* **344**, 563–570

PART 5

Practical application of secondary prevention strategies

Chapter 6

Practical application of secondary prevention after acute coronary syndromes

Adam D Timmis and Sheila Ryan

Introduction

Effective secondary prevention for patients with acute coronary syndromes requires an appropriate infrastructure for its delivery and success. This involves dedicated cardiologists and cardiac nurses to review patients in the coronary care unit (CCU), prescribe drugs of proven value for secondary prevention and deliver lifestyle advice and support. Staff and facilities are also required for outpatient review, rehabilitation courses, home visits and long-term support.

Drugs for secondary prevention

The prescription of aspirin, β blockers, angiotensin-converting enzyme (ACE) inhibitors and statins is the least demanding of all secondary prevention measures, yet doctors often fail in this simple task. The reasons for failure are complex but may include fundamental misunderstanding of the evidence base, particularly when coronary care is put in the hands of the general physicians. Thus, heart failure, diabetes, chronic obstructive pulmonary disease (COPD), peripheral vascular disease and advanced age may still be seen as contraindications to β blockers, while ACE inhibitors are often restricted to patients with severe heart failure. Large numbers of dyslipidaemic patients continue to leave hospital untreated and fibrates, in particular, are almost never prescribed even when hypertriglyceridaemia is documented.

At Newham, all patients with acute coronary syndromes are supervised by cardiologists during treatment in the CCU. A recent audit of discharge medications for patients with acute myocardial infarction showed prescription rates as follows: aspirin 96 per cent, β blockers 62 per cent, ACE inhibitors 44 per cent, lipid-lowering drugs 55 per cent. These data provide no grounds for complacency, but they are better than recent data reported from a unit run by general physicians: aspirin 89 per cent, β blockers 52 per cent, ACE inhibitors 11 per cent, lipid-lowering drugs 12 per cent (Holt *et al.* 1999). The message, now emphasised within the National Service Framework (NSF) document, is clear: prescription rates of these drugs must be improved if further reductions in coronary mortality are to be achieved. The NSF has set an 80 per cent target prescription rate and for this to be achieved it will be essential to ensure specialist cardiac involvement in the CCU management of all patients with acute coronary syndromes.

Mechanisms for early review of all secondary prevention drugs within specialist clinics are often not in place but are necessary if treatment is to be maximised and therapeutic dosage achieved. At Newham a secondary prevention clinic was established some years ago and early audit confirmed its success for reviewing drug therapy and modifying risk factors, particularly smoking, blood presure and lipids. Initially, the clinic was doctor-led but has now been replaced by a nurse-led clinic with no loss of effectiveness. A specialist smoking clinic has also been set up, run by a dedicated psychologist, and smokers unable to quit are encouraged to attend. Again, early audit points to the value of the clinic for achieving long-term smoking cessation in resistant cases.

An acute cardiac event causes distress and impaired quality of life for patients and their relatives (Mayou *et al.* 1976, 1978). These reactions are often unrelated to the severity and extent of the heart disease.

Secondary prevention packages which include cardiac rehabilitation can help support and deal with these issues, address modifiable risk factors as well as ensuring that secondary prevention medications are optimised. Rehabilitation should start on day 1 with rehabilitation nurses being a member of the acute cardiac team.

The National Service Framework states that 'The early stages of rehabilitation should be an integral component of the acute service that they provide'.

Cardiac rehabilitation, where possible, aims to stop further progression of coronary heart disease (CHD). The World Health Organization (WHO) in 1993 defined cardiac rehabilitation as 'The rehabilitation of cardiac patients is the sum of activities required to influence favourably the underlying cause of the disease, as well as the best possible physical, mental and social conditions, so that they may, by their own efforts preserve or resume when lost, as normal a place as possible in the community. Rehabilitation cannot be regarded as an isolated form of therapy but must be integrated with the whole treatment of which it forms only one facet' (WHO 1993).

Practical application in Newham

Newham is situated to the east of London with a population of 228,000 people. It is an area high in socio-economic deprivation with a large diversity of ethnic groups especially from south Asia. This results in a higher than national burden of coronary heart disease.

Newham's cardiac rehabilitation service is funded by the community trust and works alongside cardiology and nursing colleagues from the acute trust.

Rehabilitation following an acute cardiac event is offered in four phases.

Phase 1 (in-patient)

In Newham it has been recognised that, with the stay following the acute event being an average of five days, realistically this can only be the beginning of any change required in attitude, adjustment and lifestyle.

Risk factor assessment and advice while in hospital must be supported by easy to understand leaflets, which need to be made available in languages that reflect the needs of the local population. With 40 per cent of those referred not having English as their first language, Newham has booklets available in ten different languages and has an excellent health advocacy department which helps in the delivery of the service.

Phase 2 (initial out-patient)

The need for support for both the patient and their family often increases after discharge. As many as 20 per cent are said to be depressed at one month, and if left untreated 20–35 per cent remain depressed at one year (Lloyd & Cawley 1983). The need therefore is to continue the service by offering a home visit within 1–2 weeks after discharge. It is also said that patients forget information offered to them in hospital because of distress (Liddy & Crowley 1985). The early days have been described as the most critical for making the patient receptive to changes in lifestyle (Squires *et al.* 1990).

This visit at home by a specialist nurse deals with:

- patients' and families' feeling of uncertainty;
- reinforcement of advice;
- ensuring compliance of medication;
- detecting any complications.

Table 6.1 shows the actions required following such a home visit. It undoubtedly prevents many further admissions by the early detection and actions of the team.

Patients are also issued at the home visit with a hand-held record (Figure 6.1) – a simple tool to aid and share information. It also empowers patients by allowing them to know more about their condition and parameters such as cholesterol, blood pressure, pulse, body mass index (BMI) and prescribed medication.

Nurses are in an ideal position to continue to offer ongoing support and motivation to clients and their families in the community, and a nurse-led coronary secondary prevention clinic can facilitate this process.

Table 6.1 Actions following home visits (April 1999–March 2000). Total visits = 380

- 65 needed change to prescribed medication.
- 33 needed referrals to other professionals (dietitian, health visitors, district nurses, GPs, occupational therapists, benefit advice, social worker)
- 25 required a further home visit
- 13 referred back to cardiologist due to change in their clinical condition (increase in angina, BP, etc.)
- 6 required admission to hospital

RISK FACTORS (✔) where applicable	Y	N	**PERSONAL TARGETS**
Smoking (past or present)	☐	☐	
Little exercise	☐	☐	
Family History (Under 60 years)	☐	☐	
High Blood Pressure	☐	☐	
High Cholesterol	☐	☐	
Diabetes	☐	☐	

♥ **RISK FACTOR TRACKING RECORD** ♥

DATE	BLOOD PRESSURE	PULSE	CHOLESTEROL	SMOKING	WEIGHT	BMI	COMMENTS/RECHECK DATE

Figure 6.1 Example of patient hand-held record.

Lifestyle advice continues to follow a patient-centred approach:

- clarifying and gaining patients views as to their readiness to change;
- exploring and explaining the reasons for the need to change;
- agreeing goals between the patient and the nurse; if necessary giving information or referring on to local resources (such as local smoking cessation clinics);
- offering support to achieve and maintain those goals.

Also, at the time of this consultation, the following would be recorded and acted upon:

- blood pressure,
- pulse,
- body mass index,
- medication compliance,
- symptoms since discharge (chest pain, SOB, ankle swelling, etc.).

In an audit of 51 patients in 1997, 97 per cent of patients reported a reduction in anxiety following their attendance at this clinic.

Phase 3 (six week, twice-weekly classes)

Cardiac rehabilitation is known to be effective when it includes education, psychological support and exercise. These classes are co-ordinated and run by the core team but include input from a multidisciplinary team, which includes cardiologists, CCU nurses, dietitians, pharmacists, psychologists and past service users.

The model of group activity can be difficult to deliver when up to 50 per cent of the group do not share the same language. It is vital to try to ensure that non-English clients' needs are addressed by translation of written literature, using health advocates or interpreters and, where possible, translating health-related information on to audio-tapes so patients may listen in their own language.

For those too frail to attend, a home rehabilitation package should be available looking at individual risk factors in the patient's home.

Phase 4 (long term)

In the longer term, community-based exercise groups at local leisure centres, walking groups around the local area as well as patient-led support groups can help with the process of long-term behavioural change and maintain the benefits of increased physical activity.

Conclusion

Secondary prevention provides the most effective method of reducing mortality and morbidity from CHD, and treatments directed at controlling blood pressure, correcting raised cholesterol and modifying ventricular remodelling, together with addressing lifestyle issues such as smoking, represent the most vital therapeutic interventions in cardiological practice.

The recent National Service Framework document has recognised the importance of these simple measures and has set largely reasonable treatment targets, against which our performance as cardiologists and rehabilitation specialist nurses will in future be judged.

References

Holt ND, Johnson A, Davies AA, Stewart M, Hall JA, De Belder M. (1999). Secondary prevention in coronary artery disease: Have we moved on from ASPIRE? *British Journal of Cardiology* **6**, 584–588

Liddy GK & Crowley (1985). Do MI patients have the information they need for the recovery phase at home ? *Home Care Nurses* **5**, 19–25

Lloyd GG & Cawley RH (1983). Distress or illness? A study of psychological symptoms after myocardial infarction. *British Journal of Psychiatry* **142**, 120–125

Mayou R, Foster A, Williamson B (1976). Attitudes and advice after myocardial infarction. *British Medical Journal* **i**, 1577–1579

Mayou R, Foster A, Williamson B (1978). The psychological and social effects of myocardial infarction on wives. *British Medical Journal* **i**, 699–701

Squires RW, Gau GT, Miller TD (1990). Cardiovascular rehabilitation: status 1990. *Mayo Clinic Proceedings* **65**, 731–755

World Health Organization (1993). *Needs and Action Priorities in Cardiac Rehabilitation & Secondary Prevention in Patients with Coronary Heart Disease.* Geneva: WHO

Chapter 7

Practical application of secondary prevention for exertional angina in the hospital setting

David Wood

Introduction

Cardiac rehabilitation programmes are traditionally offered to patients following a myocardial infarction or after cardiac surgery, but unusually for those with exertional angina. A community register of coronary heart disease (CHD) in Bromley in south-east London shows exertional angina to be the most common first symptomatic presentation of coronary artery disease, representing approximately half of all new patients in this population (Sutcliffe *et al.* 1999). Such patients are at increased risk of progressing to myocardial infarction and coronary death, a risk that appears to be greatest in the first year following medical diagnosis (Ghandi *et al.* 1995). There is therefore considerable potential to reduce the risk of progression to unstable angina, myocardial infarction and coronary death through effective lifestyle, risk factor and therapeutic interventions. A cardiac prevention and rehabilitation service could provide such a comprehensive intervention programme for angina patients.

The joint British societies' recommendations on coronary prevention advocate that care of coronary patients should embrace all aspects of cardiac prevention and rehabilitation and such a service is made available to all patients with coronary disease, including those with exertional angina (British Cardiac Society *et al.* 2000). In the National Service Framework (NSF) for CHD, cardiac rehabilitation is seen as an integral component of the acute stages of care of both coronary disease and secondary prevention (Department of Health 2000). Once hospitals have an effective cardiac prevention and rehabilitation programme for patients who have survived a myocardial infarction, or undergone coronary revascularisation, the NSF recommends that this service be extended to people with other manifestations of coronary disease, including angina. The advent of rapid access chest pain clinics (RACPCs) nationwide (Department of Health 2000) now means that patients presenting with new angina in the community will eventually all be assessed at hospital, and this service will facilitate recruitment to a hospital-based cardiac prevention and rehabilitation programme. The NSF for CHD on stable angina has set the standard that patients with symptoms of angina or suspected angina should receive appropriate investigation and treatment to relieve pain and reduce their risk of coronary events. General practitioners must have access to specialist assessment within two weeks of referral, and the preferred model is the RACPC. In this way, patients will have ready access to a specialist opinion, supported by specialist investigations, and those at high risk can proceed to coronary angiography and, where appropriate, revascularisation. As part of this assessment it is important to address lifestyle and other risk factors together with the use of prophylactic drug therapies.

The scientific evidence for secondary prevention of coronary disease, reviewed in the joint British societies' original report (Wood *et al.* 1998), provides a strong basis for lifestyle interventions (Law & Tang 1995), aspirin (Antiplatelet Trialist Collaboration 1994), post-myocardial infarction treatment with β blockers (Yusuf *et al.* 1985) and angiotensin-converting enzyme (ACE) inhibitors (Acute Infarction Ramipril Efficacy [AIRE] Investigators 1993), lipid-lowering (statins) drugs (Scandinavian Simvastatin Survival Study 1994; Sacks *et al.* 1996; Long-Term Intervention with Pravastatin in Ischaemic Disease [LIPID] Study Group 1998) and revascularisation (Yusuf *et al.* 1994) on prognostic grounds. Where available this evidence also applies to patients with angina (aspirin) (Antiplatelet Trialists Collaboration 1994) and lipid-lowering (Scandinavian Simvastatin Survival Study 1994) treatment, and therefore lifestyle and risk factor management is recommended to be the same for all manifestations of coronary artery disease – acute myocardial infarction, unstable angina and exertional angina. Lifestyle, risk factor and therapeutic targets recommended in the joint British societies' report have been adopted by the NSF for CHD (Department of Health 2000). The report recommended lifestyle intervention to discontinue smoking, make healthier food choices, increase aerobic exercise and moderate alcohol consumption by all patients with CHD, and the involvement of the whole family is emphasised. Rigorous control of blood pressure, lipids and glucose is recommended with the following treatment targets:

- BP < 140 mmHg systolic and < 85 mmHg diastolic;
- total cholesterol < 5.0 mmol/l (LDL-cholesterol < 3.0 mmol/l);
- diabetes mellitus should be optimally controlled with insulin during and immediately after an acute myocardial infarction (MI), and blood pressure reduced to < 130 mmHg systolic and < 80 mmHg diastolic.

Cardioprotective drug therapy should be considered and prescribed in coronary patients:

- aspirin for all patients
- β blockers at the doses prescribed in the clinical trials following MI, particularly in high-risk patients, and for at least three years
- cholesterol-lowering therapy (statins) at the doses prescribed in the clinical trials
- ACE inhibitors at the doses prescribed in the clinical trials for patients with symptoms or signs of heart failure at the time of MI, or in those with persistent left ventricular systolic dysfunction (ejection fraction < 40%)

- anticoagulants for patients at risk of systemic embolisation with large anterior infarctions, severe heart failure, left ventricular aneurysm or paroxysmal tachyarrhythmias.

Since these recommendations were published in 1998, the evidence for platelet modification therapy is further strengthened by the results of a systematic review of thienopyridine derivatives (ticlopidine, clopidogrel) versus aspirin (Hankey *et al.* 2001). Thienopyridines are significantly more effective at reducing the risk of a serious vascular event, including stroke, with a lower risk of gastrointestinal haemorrhage compared with aspirin. At present aspirin is still the preferred first-line anti-platelet drug, but clopidogrel should be considered as alternative long-term treatment (CAPRIE Steering Committee 1996) if aspirin is not tolerated, or there is an increased risk of bleeding. The evidence for β blockade after myocardial infarction is reinforced by a systematic review (Freemantle 1999). The long-term evidence for ACE inhibitors after an MI complicated by heart failure is strengthened by the continuing survival benefit over seven years after the initial event (Hall *et al.* 1997). A systematic overview of ACE inhibitor therapy started during acute MI provides additional evidence of a short-term mortality benefit, particularly in patients with an anterior MI and in those at increased risk of death (ACE Inhibitor Myocardial Infarction Collaborative Group 1998). The indications for an ACE inhibitor have been further extended beyond patients with heart failure, or left ventricular systolic dysfunction, by the results of the HOPE trial (Yusuf *et al.* 2000). Ramipril reduced the risk of all-cause deaths, cardiovascular deaths, MI, stroke, heart failure and complications related to diabetes in patients with vascular disease or diabetes and with preserved ventricular function. So, for coronary patients, it is now also appropriate to use ACE inhibitors in those who are without heart failure or a low ejection fraction.

In addition to offering a cardiac prevention and rehabilitation service to all coronary patients, the joint British societies' report (Wood *et al.* 1998) recommended integration of patient care between hospital and general practice, through common clinical protocols, to ensure optimal long-term lifestyle, risk factor and therapeutic management. Screening of first-degree blood relatives (principally siblings and off-spring aged 18 years or older) of patients with premature CHD (men < 55 years and women < 65 years) is encouraged and, in the context of familial dyslipidaemias, is considered essential. Auditing the impact of common clinical protocols between hospital and general practice for coronary patient management is strongly recommended.

Bromley 'Changes for Life' programme

A cardiac prevention and rehabilitation programme was established at Bromley Hospitals NHS Trust, south-east London, in October 1997, for all first presentations of CHD in the district and the main results of this programme are currently being published (Fox *et al.* 2001). This service replaced a small traditional cardiac rehabilitation programme restricted to selected patients after MI or coronary surgery. The objective was to achieve defined lifestyle, risk factor and therapeutic targets comparable to those subsequently published by the joint British societies' report and the NSF on CHD. Specifically, the lifestyle objectives were to help patients and families quit tobacco, make healthier food choices and be more physically active. In addition, the following targets were set: body mass index (BMI) < 25 kg/m^2, blood pressure $< 140/90$ mmHg, total cholesterol < 4.8 mmol/l and optimal glycaemic control of diabetes. Therapeutic targets were: aspirin for all patients; β blockers following MI (and to be prescribed as first-line antianginal therapy or as first-choice antihypertensive agent) and lipid-lowering therapy in the form of a statin to achieve a cholesterol target of < 4.8 mmol/l – a target defined at the start of the programme from the post-hoc analysis of the CARE trial (Sacks *et al.* 1996). ACE inhibitors were being used for post-infarction patients with heart failure based on the AIRE criteria (AIRE Investigators 1993), but there was no other specific target for ACE inhibitor use in the programme. Screening of family members, both partners and first-degree relatives, was an integral part of this service.

Setting

Bromley Health Authority (population 292,000) is served by 151 GPs in 59 practices. Bromley Hospital (with the Cardiac Care Unit [CCU] and Accident & Emergency Department [A&E]) and Farnborough Hospital provide secondary cardiac care, whereas the specialist cardiac centres at King's College Hospital, the Royal Brompton and Harefield and St Thomas's Hospital provided tertiary care. An RACPC was opened at Bromley Hospital in 1996 to which GPs could refer all patients presenting for the first time with symptoms of exertional angina, but with no past medical history of coronary disease. Therefore, the cardiology department at Bromley Hospital provided direct access to hospital care for all coronary patients, either through A&E or by referral to the RACPC.

The 'Changes for Life' programme

This cardiac prevention and rehabilitation programme (Figure 7.1) was led by a cardiologist and run by two full-time cardiac prevention nurses, a physiotherapist (one-fifth time) and a dietitian (one-fifth time) with advice from other healthcare professionals.

Recruitment

Patients admitted to hospital with acute myocardial infarction or unstable angina were identified by the cardiac prevention nurses through CCU, the cardiology ward or other wards in the two hospitals, and offered a place on the programme. This nurse then remained as the patients' primary nurse throughout the programme. If the

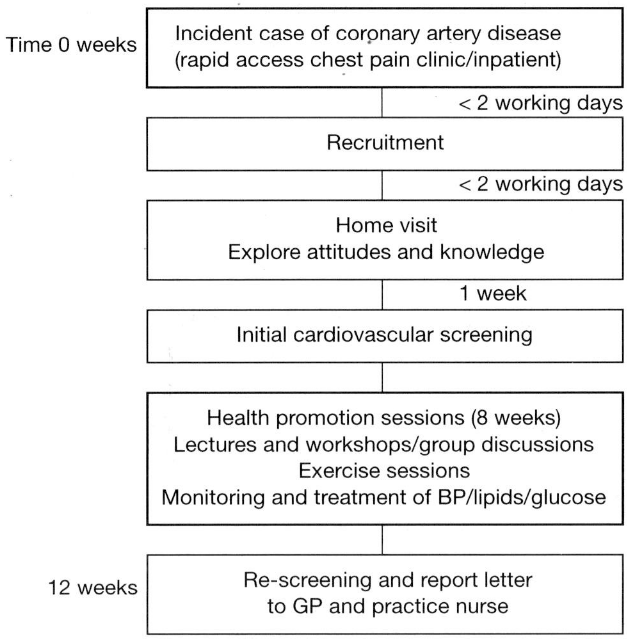

Figure 7.1 The Bromley 'Changes for Life' programme

patient agreed to participate, a home visit followed usually within two working days of hospital discharge. Patients with exertional angina identified through the RACPC were contacted by a cardiac prevention nurse to arrange a home visit, also usually within two working days of being diagnosed in the RACPC. At the home visit the patient was given a copy of the 'Cardiofax' (a filo-fax format) containing information about the 'Changes for Life' programme, the causes of coronary disease, lifestyle, other risk factors and other documentation. The patient's partner was encouraged to be present at this home visit and at all subsequent meetings and cardiovascular screening was offered to partners and offspring (≥ 16 years old).

Initial cardiovascular screening

The initial cardiovascular screening of patients and family members included an assessment of lifestyle (smoking, diet and physical activity), height and weight (to calculate BMI: weight [kg]/height^2 [m^2]), blood pressure (two readings at rest), random cholesterol and fasting lipids, blood glucose and pharmacological treatment. A dietitian was responsible for individual or family dietary assessment and advice. Lifestyle changes were negotiated and targets discussed as already described. A policy of evidence-based prescribing was followed, using drug doses as prescribed in those clinical trials that have reported both efficacy, in terms of reducing clinical events, and long-term safety.

After this initial cardiovascular screening, a multidisciplinary health promotion programme took place over eight weekly sessions, usually starting within a week or so of hospital discharge or RACPC assessment. Behavioural change in the programme was based on the Prochaska and DiClemente cycle of change, promoted by the Health Education Authority, encouraging thinking about change, preparing to change, making changes, maintaining changes and addressing relapse (Prochaska & DiClemente 1986). The cardiac prevention nurses, and other members of the 'Changes for Life' team, were all instructed in this approach by a clinical psychologist. The programme covered CHD risk factors, family support and change, stopping smoking, diet and weight, physical activity, stress management, treatment and the role of support groups. A group discussion was held one week after each lecture to allow participants time to assimilate facts and formulate questions. At each weekly session, supervised exercise for one hour was led by a physiotherapist and included a warm-up period, three groups of exercises and a cool-down period. At the end of the eight weekly sessions each patient was given an individual exercise plan by the physiotherapist.

Protocol-based assessment and management of blood pressure, blood lipids and glucose was followed by the nurses. Blood pressure was monitored twice a week and the target for blood pressure was < 140/90 mmHg. A physician was responsible for optimising antihypertensive treatment as required. Patients who had had an acute coronary syndrome were started immediately on a statin in hospital if the initial random cholesterol concentration was > 6 mmol/l. If the cholesterol was < 6.0 mmol/l this was repeated eight weeks later on three separate occasions (including one fasting lipid profile). If the average total cholesterol was > 4.8 mmol/l a physician prescribed a statin. For all other coronary patients, regardless of their initial cholesterol concentration, the same outpatient protocol was followed: three separate lipid measurements (including one fasting) during the programme, and physician-initiated treatment if the average concentration was > 4.8 mmol/l. Patients with a random glucose concentration of > 6.7 mmol/l had a measurement of glycated haemoglobin (HbA1c). If this was abnormal they were referred to a diabetes specialist for further evaluation and management.

The patients' symptoms and medical status were monitored by the nurses throughout the programme with referral back as required to the consultant physician responsible for their care.

Re-screening

On completion of the health promotion sessions, patients and screened family members were re-screened for lifestyle, blood pressure, cholesterol, glucose and use of drug treatment. An electronic report was prepared and sent to the patient's GP and a practice nurse, giving results in relation to defined lifestyle, risk factor and therapeutic targets, and what further action, if any, was required.

One-year follow-up

Patients were sent a letter inviting them for interview one year after completing the programme. This included questions on lifestyle and drug treatment, and measurements of BMI, blood pressure (two readings at rest) and non-fasting total cholesterol.

The programme's results

Between October 1997 and December 1998, 194 coronary patients were identified and 158 recruited to the programme (response rate 82%): 87 (55%) had exertional angina, 50 (32%) acute MI, 9 (6%) unstable angina and 12 (7%) other diagnoses (e.g. recent myocardial infarction). The majority of angina patients were recruited through the RACPC. Mean age of all patients was 65 years (range 31–90 years): men 64 years, women 66 years. Of the patients recruited 148 (94%) received a home visit and 133 (84%) attended the initial cardiovascular screening in hospital and entered the rolling programme of health promotion sessions. One hundred and thirteen (72%) completed these sessions and 102 (65%) attended for re-screening at 12 weeks and a report was sent to their GP and practice nurse. Completion of the programme did not differ significantly by diagnosis, place of recruitment (in-patient, RACPC or other), age or sex. Of the patients who participated in the programme, 96 (72%) attended for the one-year follow-up, which was completed in December 1999.

Lifestyle characteristics, other risk factors and use of drug therapies at initial screening, final re-screening and one-year follow-up for patients with exertional angina are shown in Table 7.1 and for those with acute coronary syndromes (ACS – acute MI and unstable angina) in Table 7.2. Patients with other coronary diagnoses, e.g. recent MI, are included in the ACS group. The vast majority of angina and ACS patients were not smoking at the start of the programme and this was sustained at one-year follow-up. There were more overweight and obese angina patients compared with those with ACS at both the beginning and the end of the programme. The majority of all coronary patients had not reached the target BMI of < 25 kg/m^2 at one year. Over two-thirds of angina and ACS patients had achieved the blood pressure goal of $< 140/90$ mmHg at the end of the programme and, although these proportions had fallen slightly at one year, most of the patients had still maintained this target. A majority of both angina and ACS patients had also achieved the current national target cholesterol of < 5.0 mmol/l (Department of Health 2000) at the end of the programme and at one year. As many ACS patients had their treatment initiated in hospital, 54 per cent had already achieved the cholesterol target by the start of the programme, unlike those with angina. Only 20 per cent of angina patients had reached the cholesterol target at the same point in the programme but this increased to 59 per cent at the end of the programme.

Table 7.1 Cardiovascular risk factors in patients with exertional angina at initial screening examination, re-screening at the end of the programme and 1-year follow-up

Characteristic	*All patients screened*	*Patients who took part in the health promotion programme*		
	Initial screening (n = 77)	*Initial screening*[a] *(n = 58)*	*Re-screening (n = 58)*	*1-year follow-up (n = 56)*
Non-smoking status (%)	86	88	91	91
Weight (kg) [mean(SD)]	78.9(12.0)	77.8(10.2)	77.8(10.6)	78.6(11.3)
Body mass index (kg/m^2) [mean(SD)]	28.2(4.6)	27.9(4.6)	27.9(4.6)	28.0(4.5)
Percentage BMI < 25 kg/m^2	24	26	28	23
Systolic BP (mmHg) [mean(SD)]	136(21)	135(21)	136(16)	134(18)
Diastolic BP (mmHg) [mean(SD)]	79(12)	79(12)	77(10)	77(11)
Percentage < 140/90 mmHg	57	58	67	57
Total cholesterol (mmol/l) [mean(SD)]	5.6(1.1)	5.6(1.1)	4.7(0.9)	4.9(1.0)
Percentage < 4.8 mmol/l	21	20	59	54
Aspirin therapy (%)	96	95	95	88
β-Blocker therapy (%)	58	62	59	45
Lipid-lowering therapy (%)	23	24	62	55

[a]Initial screening results for those attending for re-screening.

Table 7.2 Cardiovascular risk factors in patients with acute coronary syndromes at initial screening examination, re-screening at the end of the programme and 1-year follow-up

	All patients screened	*Patients who took part in the health promotion programme*		
Characteristic	*Initial screening (n = 56)*	*Initial screening[a] (n = 44)*	*Re-screening (n = 44)*	*1-year follow-up (n = 39)*
Non-smoking status (%)	89	89	93	92
Weight (kg) [mean(SD)]	76.3(13.6)	76.6(13.8)	76.1(13.8)	76.4(14.0)
Body mass index (kg/m^2) [mean(SD)]	27.0(4.7)	26.9(4.7)	26.6(4.6)	26.6(4.3)
Percentage BMI < 25 kg/m^2	38	40	41	37
Systolic BP (mmHg) [mean(SD)]	129(18)	129(17)	131(22)	134(23)
Diastolic BP (mmHg) [mean(SD)]	77(11)	78(13)	77(11)	79(12)
Percentage < 140/90 mmHg	75	75	73	59
Total cholesterol (mmol/l) [mean(SD)]	4.9(1.0)	4.8(1.0)	4.6(0.8)	5.0(1.1)
Percentage < 4.8 mmol/l	52	54	66	54
Aspirin therapy (%)	100	100	98	90
β-Blocker therapy (%)	61	68	66	54
Lipid-lowering therapy (%)	52	55	66	56

[a]Initial screening results for those attending for re-screening.

The proportions of patients with angina and ACS achieving the cholesterol target by the end of the programme was therefore similar, and at one year proportions were identical. The use of aspirin and β blockers in angina and ACS patients was similar. Of ACS patients, 55 per cent were already taking lipid-lowering therapy at the start of the programme, in contrast to 24 per cent of those with angina. At the end of the programme there was little difference, and at one year no difference, in the use of lipid-lowering therapy between these diagnostic groups. However, there was a decrease in the use of all three classes of prophylactic drug therapies for both angina and ACS patients at one year. After taking account of differences in baseline values between exertional angina and ACS patients, there was no evidence of any statistically significant differences between these diagnostic groups (nor when comparing angina with the acute MI group alone) for any of the lifestyle, risk factor or therapeutic targets on completion of the programme, or at one-year follow-up.

Commentary

The prevention of CHD is a government priority and cardiac rehabilitation is one key element of the NSF for CHD (Department of Health 2000). The joint British societies' recommendations on coronary prevention in clinical practice define patients with established coronary disease, or other atherosclerotic disease, as the top priority (British Cardiac Society *et al.* 2000). In hospitals it is recommended that care of such patients embrace all aspects of cardiac prevention and rehabilitation, and be offered to all coronary patients, not just those following an MI or revascularisation (Wood *et al.* 1998). Providing such a service in the NSF for CHD is recognised as a hospital trust responsibility (Department of Health 2000).

The cardiology service developed at Bromley Hospitals NHS Trust between 1996 and 1998 provided a complete spectrum of care from rapid chest pain assessment in an RACPC, to CCU and in-patient care, and then on to cardiac prevention and rehabilitation. This innovative service anticipated the key elements of the NSF on CHD (Department of Health 2000) by setting new standards of care for all patients with coronary artery disease – those with angina as well as acute coronary syndromes – in the community. The Bromley 'Changes for Life' programme shows how a comprehensive cardiac prevention and rehabilitation service can be organised for all such patients, including those with exertional angina. The programme set targets for lifestyle, risk factor management and the use of prophylactic drug therapies, and these were achieved with equal success by patients with exertional angina and acute coronary syndromes. Although these results are not sustained in both diagnostic groups at one year, the majority of patients were still below the risk factor targets at this point, and these results are a substantial improvement on those reported from the Action on Secondary Prevention by Intervention to Reduce Events (ASPIRE) study (ASPIRE Steering Group 1996) in the early 1990s.

In the ASPIRE survey 2,583 coronary patients aged 70 years or over were examined from a random sample of 24 specialist cardiac centres and district general hospitals in the UK (ASPIRE Steering Group 1996). The patients were drawn from four diagnostic categories: coronary artery surgery, percutaneous coronary intervention, acute MI and myocardial ischaemia without evidence of infarction. At interview (at least six months after their hospital admission), 19 per cent were smoking cigarettes and 72 per cent were overweight (BMI ≥ 25 kg/m^2), of whom 28 per cent were obese (BMI ≥ 30 kg/ m^2). Fifty per cent had a diastolic blood pressure ≥ 90 mmHg and/or a systolic pressure ≥ 140 mmHg; 82 per cent had a blood cholesterol ≥ 5.0 mmol/l. Prescribed prophylactic drug therapies were as follows: aspirin (86%), β blockers (38%) and lipid-lowering drugs (19%). Therefore, the 'Changes for Life' programme has achieved a better lifestyle profile, at least for smoking, and more effective control of both blood pressure and cholesterol. The use of prophylactic drug therapies has also increased, especially for lipid-lowering drugs in the form of statins.

The Bromley 'Changes for Life' programme had several specific features. First, all patients with coronary disease were eligible for the programme, not just those presenting with MI or after revascularisation. Second, the patient's cardiological management was completely integrated with all aspects of secondary prevention, whether admitted to the CCU or the wards or assessed in the RACPC. The cardiac prevention nurses were part of the cardiology team, which as a whole focused on risk factors and prophylactic therapeutic management. Patients were actively recruited to the programme by the specialist nurses immediately after diagnosis, rather than referred, and this is the most likely explanation for the high recruitment rate compared with other programmes (Cooper *et al.* 1999). The RACPC facilitated the recruitment of angina patients. This new cardiology service ensured that almost all patients presenting with exertional angina in the community were appropriately assessed by a cardiologist, and most then entered the cardiac prevention and rehabilitation programme. A similarly high recruitment rate was also seen for acute MI and unstable angina, and there were no differences in recruitment rates by age or sex. Patients were visited at home and partner and blood relative involvement was encouraged in the initial cardiovascular screening in hospital, attendance at health promotion sessions and the final reassessment, before being discharged to the general practice. The involvement of the whole family is likely to increase the chances of lifestyle targets being achieved (Sackett *et al.* 1975; Pyke *et al.* 1997). The immediate blood relatives can also be screened for cardiovascular risk factors, which facilitates the detection of familial dyslipidaemias.

Although the joint British societies' recommendations were not published at the time this programme was set up, defined lifestyle, risk factor and therapeutic targets were set. The blood pressure target of < 140/90 mmHg was not as rigorous as the current target of < 140/85 mmHg, and no separate blood pressure target was set for patients with diabetes mellitus. The cholesterol target in this programme of < 4.8 mmol/l was slightly lower than the current national cholesterol target of < 5.0 mmol/l. These targets, together with nurse-led protocols for blood pressure and lipid management, ensured more effective management of patients compared with ASPIRE (ASPIRE Steering Group 1996). The re-screening at the end of the programme reinforced these targets, and highlighted those not achieved on discharge to general practice. Continuity of care was helped by sending an electronic report to both the GP and the practice nurse, and arranging a follow-up appointment with the practice, shortly after leaving the programme.

Conclusions

A comprehensive cardiac prevention and rehabilitation programme can be offered to all patients presenting for the first time with coronary artery disease. The development of rapid access chest pain clinics in hospitals across the country will ensure that most patients with exertional angina are assessed in hospital, thus facilitating their recruitment to such hospital-based programmes. Patients with exertional angina could eventually constitute the majority of patients in these programmes. A high recruitment of patients with exertional angina can be achieved, similar to that for MI. Lifestyle, risk factor and therapeutic targets can be successfully reached in the majority of patients with exertional angina, with no difference in outcome for angina compared with ACSs. This programme substantially improved the standard of care found in ASPIRE, and patients who achieve and maintain lifestyle, risk factor and therapeutic targets over the long term can expect a corresponding reduction in coronary morbidity and mortality.

References

Acute Infarction Ramipril Efficacy (AIRE) Investigators (1993). Effects of ramipril on morbidity and mortality of survivors of acute myocardial infarction with clinical evidence of heart failure. *The Lancet* **342**, 821–828

Antiplatelet Trialists' Collaboration (1994). Collaborative overview of randomises trials of antiplatelet therapy. 1. Prevention of death, myocardial infarction and stroke by prolonged antiplatelet therapy in various categories of patients. *British Medical Journal* **308**, 81–106

Aspire Steering Group (1996). A British Cardiac Society survey of the potential for the secondary prevention of coronary disease: ASPIRE (action on secondary prevention through intervention to reduce events). Principal results. *Heart* **75**, 334–342

British Cardiac Society, British Hyperlipidaemia Association, British Hypertension Society, British Diabetic Association (2000). Joint British recommendations on prevention of coronary heart disease in clinical practice: summary. *British Medical Journal* **320**, 705–708

CAPRIE Steering Committee (1996). A randomised, blinded, trial of clopidogrel versus aspirin in patients at risk of ischaemic events (CAPRIE). *The Lancet* **348**, 1329–1339

Cooper R, Lloyd G, Weinman J *et al.* (1999). Why patients do not attend cardiac rehabilitation: role of intentions and illness beliefs. *Heart* **82**, 234–236

Department of Health (2000). *The National Service Framework for Coronary Heart Disease.* London: HMSO

Fox KF, Nutall M, Wood DA *et al.* (2001). A cardiac prevention and rehabilitation programme for all patients at first presentation with coronary artery disease. *Heart* **85**, 533–538

Freemantle N, Cleland J, Young P, Mason J, Harrison J (1999). Beta blockade after myocardial infarction: Systematic review and meta regression analysis. *British Medical Journal* **318**, 1730–1737

Ghandi MM, Lampe F, Wood DA (1995). Incidence, clinical characteristics and short-term prognosis of angina pectoris. *Heart* **73**, 193–198

Hall AS, Murray GD, Ball SG (1997). Follow-up study of patients randomly allocated ramipril or placebo for heart failure after acute myocardial infarction: AIRE Extension (AIREX) Study. Acute Infarction Ramipril Efficacy. *The Lancet* **349**, 1493–1497

Hankey GJ, Sudlow CLM, Dunbabin DW (2001). Thienopyridine derivatives (ticlopidine, clopidogrel) versus aspirin for preventing stroke and other serious vascular events in high vascular risk patients. (Cochrane Review). In *The Cochrane Library, Issue 1, 2001.* Oxford: Update Software

Law M & Tang JL (1995). An analysis of the effectiveness of interventions intended to help people stop smoking. *Archives of Internal Medicine* **155**, 1933–1941

Long-term Intervention with Pravastatin in Ischaemic Disease (LIPID) Study Group (1998). Prevention of cardiovascular events and death with pravastatin in patients with coronary heart disease and a broad range of initial cholesterol levels. *New England Journal of Medicine* **339**, 1349–1357

Prochaska JO & DiClemente CC (1986). Toward a comprehensive model of change. In *Treating Addictive Behaviour: Processes of change*. New York: Plenum Press, pp 3–27

Pyke SDM, Wood DA, Kinmouth AL *et al.* (1997). Changes in coronary risk and risk factor levels in couples following lifestyle intervention: the British family heart study. *Archives of Family Medicine* **6**, 3254–3260

Sackett DL, Anderson GD, Milner R *et al.* (1975). Concordance for coronary risk factors among spouses. *Circulation* **52**, 589–595

Sacks FM, Pfeffer MA, Moye LA *et al.* (1996). The effect of pravastatin on coronary events after myocardial infarction in patients with average lipid levels. *New England Journal of Medicine* **335**, 1001–1009

Scandinavian Simvastatin Survival Study (1994). A randomised trial of cholesterol lowering in 4444 patients with coronary heart disease: the Scandinavian simvastatin survival study (4S). *The Lancet* **344**, 1383–1389

Sutcliffe SJ, Sutcliffe AK, Wood DA (1999). The clinical incidence of fatal and non-fatal coronary heart disease in the population. *Heart* **81**, 28

Yusuf S, Peto R, Lewis J, Collins R, Sleight P (1985). Beta-blockers during and after myocardial infarction: an overview of the randomised trials. *Progress in Cardiovascular Diseases* **27**, 335–371

Yusuf S, Zucker D, Peduzzi P *et al.* (1994). Effect of coronary artery bypass graft surgery on survival: overview of 10 years results from randomised trials by the coronary artery bypass graft surgery trialists collaboration. *The Lancet* **344**, 563–570

Yusuf A, Sleight P, Pogue J, Bosch J, Davies R, Dagenais G (2000). Effects of an angiotensin-converting-enzyme inhibitor, ramipril, on cardiovascular events in high-risk patients. The Heart Outcomes Prevention Evaluation Study Investigators. *New England Journal of Medicine* **342**, 145–153

Wood DA, Durrington P, Poulter N *et al.* (1998). Joint British recommendations on prevention of coronary heart disease in clinical practice. *Heart* **80**, S1–S29

PART 6

Improving the quality of clinical services

Chapter 8

Prevention of coronary heart disease in UK Indian Asians

John C Chambers and Jaspal S Kooner

Epidemiology of coronary heart disease in Indian Asians

The population of the UK includes approximately 1.6 million people of Indian Asian descent, most of whom are first- or second-generation migrants. In UK Indian Asians, mortality from coronary heart disease (CHD) is 40 per cent higher (Balarajan 1996), and admission rates with myocardial infarction are twofold higher (Wilkinson *et al.* 1996), compared to the European white population. The increase in CHD risk is evident in each of the major Asian cultural subgroups, and is most striking in young men, among whom CHD mortality is at least twofold higher than in Europeans (Balarajan 1996). There is also loss of immunity from CHD in Indian Asian women.

Mechanisms underlying CHD in UK Indian Asians

Conventional CHD risk factors

The mechanisms underlying increased CHD mortality in UK Indian Asians are not well understood. Previous studies show that levels of cigarette smoking, blood pressure and cholesterol are not consistently raised in all Indian Asian subgroups compared to Europeans (Mckeigue *et al.* 1991). These observations have led to the belief that conventional risk factors do not contribute to the excess CHD mortality in Indian Asians. However, in comparison to Europeans, the prevalence of certain CHD risk factors is high in specific Asian subgroups (Bhopal *et al.* 1999). Thus, cigarette smoking is more common in Bangladeshis (Bhopal *et al.* 1999) and hypertension is more prevalent in Sikhs compared to Europeans (Mckeigue *et al.* 1991; Chambers *et al.* 2000a). Furthermore, previous studies indicate that serum cholesterol, blood pressure, smoking rates and body mass index are all substantially higher in migrant Indian Asians, compared to their non-migrant siblings (Bhatnagar *et al.* 1995). Classic risk factors must therefore impact on the high CHD rates in UK Indian Asians, although the precise extent to which each contributes to increased CHD risk in Asians remains unclear.

Diabetes and insulin resistance

A consistent finding in population studies is that the prevalence of diabetes is almost fourfold higher in UK Indian Asians than among European whites (Mather & Keen

1985; Mckeigue *et al.* 1991; Chambers *et al.* 2000a). Almost 20 per cent of Indian Asian men have diabetes, one-third of whom are undiagnosed (Anand *et al.* 2000; Chambers *et al.* 2000a). In addition, insulin resistance and its related metabolic abnormalities (central obesity, glucose intolerance, elevated plasma insulin, increased triglycerides, raised PAI-1 and reduced high-density lipoprotein [HDL] cholesterol) are more common among Indian Asians than Europeans (Mckeigue *et al.* 1991, 1993; Anand *et al.* 2000; Chambers *et al.* 2000a). These metabolic disturbances are increasingly recognised as risk factors for CHD, and may account for up to 70 per cent of major Q wave ECG abnormalities in Indian Asians (Mckeigue *et al.* 1993). The mechanisms underlying increased insulin resistance in UK Indian Asians remain to be determined. Findings that glucose and insulin concentrations are higher, and that HDL-cholesterol is lower, in migrant compared to non-migrant Indian Asian siblings, suggest that environmental factors contribute to these disturbances (Bhatnagar *et al.* 1995). In addition, defective insulin action is found in the asymptomatic first-degree relatives of UK Indian Asian survivors of premature myocardial infarction (MI), suggesting that a component of insulin resistance is inherited in this racial group (Kooner *et al.* 1998).

Novel risk factors for CHD

More recent studies show that concentrations of plasma homocysteine, an emerging risk factor for CHD, are higher in Indian Asians than in European whites, and suggest that homocysteine may contribute to increased CHD mortality rate in the former (Anand *et al.* 2000; Chambers *et al.* 2000a). Among Indian Asians, elevated homocysteine is accounted for by reduced levels of vitamins B_{12} and folate, compared to Europeans (Chambers *et al.* 2000a). These observations imply that the increased CHD risk in this racial group may be reduced by dietary supplementation with B vitamins. Unlike European whites, the common MTHFR C677T mutation does not contribute to increased homocysteine concentrations, and is not a risk factor for CHD in Indian Asians (Chambers *et al.* 2001). This raises the possibility that novel genetic defects, other than the MTHFR C677T mutation, may influence homocysteine metabolism in this racial group. Serum Lp(a) concentrations, influenced primarily by genetic factors (Beerwinkle *et al.* 1992), have also been reported to be higher in Indian Asians compared to Europeans, and may influence CHD risk in this racial group (Bhatnagar *et al.* 1995; Anand *et al.* 2000).

Inflammation is recognised as a central feature of atherogenesis, and may play a critical role in plaque rupture, through destabilisation of the fibrous cap (Ross 1999). C-reactive protein (CRP), the classic acute phase reactant, is a sensitive systemic marker of inflammation, increased concentrations of which have been shown to predict risk of future atherothrombotic events (Haverkate *et al.* 1997; Ridker *et al.* 2000). Recent studies indicate that CRP concentrations are higher in healthy asymptomatic Indian Asians, than in European whites (Chambers & Kooner 2000), suggesting that inflammatory mechanisms contribute to increased CHD risk in Asians. Abdominal obesity, identified in Indian Asians (Mckeigue *et al.* 1991, 1993), may have an important role, since abdominal adipose tissue is a major source of cytokines, including IL-6, an important determinant of hepatic CRP synthesis (Yudkin *et al.* 1999).

Identification of Indian Asians at increased CHD risk

Therapeutic intervention to reduce CHD events should be directed to patients with proven CHD, first-degree relatives of patients with premature CHD and individuals who are asymptomatic, but at high risk of CHD. The last include subjects with classic risk factors, central obesity, insulin resistance and associated metabolic risk factors. Identification of Indian Asians at increased CHD risk presents a major obstacle for the clinician. The Framingham study equations predict CHD risk accurately among predominantly white populations in North America (Leaverton *et al.* 1987), and have been incorporated into European and UK guidelines for the prevention of CHD (British Cardiac Society *et al.* 1998; Wood *et al.* 1998). However, recent studies indicate that the Framingham study functions underestimate CHD risk among UK Indian Asians by approximately 50 per cent (Chambers *et al.* 2000b). This may reflect the failure of these functions to take account of insulin resistance and related disturbances. A logical solution to this problem might be to lower the threshold for treatment in UK Indian Asians, although the validity of this approach remains to be determined.

Most studies support the view that insulin resistance is the key disturbance underlying increased CHD risk in UK Indian Asians. The absence of a simple, reproducible marker of insulin resistance presents an additional problem to the clinician. In practice, the combination of raised fasting triglycerides (>1.5 mmol/l), low HDL-cholesterol (<1.0 mmol/l), raised fasting glucose (>6.0mmol/l), central obesity (waist:hip girth ratio >1.0 in men and >0.85 in women) and hypertension reliably identifies insulin-resistant subjects who are likely to benefit most from risk factor modification.

Treatment of CHD risk factors in UK Indian Asians

CHD has a multifactorial aetiology, and coronary risk factors have a multiplicative effect. Effective prevention therefore requires identification and treatment of the total burden of risk, rather than single risk factors.

Conventional risk factors

Cigarette smoking rates are higher in Bangladeshi men (Bhopal *et al.* 1999) and similar in Hindu and Muslim men, compared to Europeans (Mckeigue *et al.* 1993). Cigarette smoking is one of the most important predictors of MI in Indian Asians (Pais *et al.* 1996). For individuals currently smoking ten or more cigarettes per day, the odds ratio for CHD is estimated at 6.7. Often, success on smoking cessation is greatest after the acute event. Smoking cessation may reduce CHD by about 25 per cent in Indian Asian men. Indian Asian women have very low smoking rates (Bhopal *et al.* 1999). Health promotion measures must ensure that smoking rates should not rise in second-generation UK Indian Asians.

Primary and secondary prevention studies show that cholesterol lowering reduces CHD risk even among subjects with average cholesterol levels (Sacks *et al.* 1996; Downs *et al.* 1998; The Long-term Intervention with Pravastatin in Ischaemic Disease [LIPID] Study Group 1998). In this regard, 'normal' cholesterol levels, often based on a range between 4.0 and 6.5 mmol/l, should be redefined. Total cholesterol levels have risen by almost 2 mmol/l with migration to the UK from India (Bhatnagar *et al.* 1995), and undoubtedly have a major influence on the high CHD rates in UK Indian Asians. Drug therapy to lower cholesterol should be considered in all high-risk Indian Asians, irrespective of baseline cholesterol level (Department of Health 2000). Many Indian Asians have high triglycerides and low HDL-cholesterol, and increased small dense LDL-cholesterol (Mckeigue *et al.* 1991, 1993; Anand *et al.* 2000; Chambers *et al.* 2000a). The data from clinical and metabolic studies linking mild-to-moderate hypertriglyceridaemia and low HDL-cholesterol to CHD are compelling (Assman *et al.* 1996; Harper & Jacobsen 1999; Rubins *et al.* 1999), and would favour treatment of this atherogenic phenotype. Ideally, in UK Indian Asians, the lipid profile should be similar to that for non-migrants; total cholesterol should not exceed 4.5 mmol/l, LDL-cholesterol 2.5 mmol/l, triglycerides 1.5 mmol/l and HDL-cholesterol should be higher than 1.0 mmol/l. These values are acceptable because they are similar to rural populations at low risk of CHD (Bhatnagar *et al.* 1995).

Raised blood pressure is a strong predictor of CHD (van den Hoogen *et al.* 2000) and randomised trials indicate that antihypertensive therapy is effective in reducing CHD and stroke rates (Kaplan 1992; Hansson *et al.* 1998). Observational studies show that over 40 per cent of healthy Indian Asian men have hypertension. Active attempts should be made to detect and control hypertension in these subjects. In middle-aged UK Indian Asians, blood pressure levels should probably not exceed the non-migrant blood pressure of 140/85 mmHg in men and women (Bhatnagar *et al.* 1995).

Diabetes and insulin resistance

Cardiovascular disease is the principal cause of death among patients with diabetes (Mather *et al.* 1998). The prevalence of diabetes is fourfold higher in Indian Asians than in Europeans (Mather & Keen 1985; Mckeigue *et al.* 1991; Chambers *et al.* 2000a) and diabetes is present in over 50 per cent of Indian Asian CHD patients (Chambers *et al.* 2000a). Diabetes is therefore of particular importance in this ethnic group. The results of recent studies provide unequivocal evidence that, in patients with diabetes, the incidence of myocardial infarction can be reduced by 21 per cent through rigorous blood pressure control (target: <130/80 mmHg), and by 16 per cent through tight control of blood glucose (target: fasting plasma glucose <6.0 mmol/l) (UK Prospective Diabetes Study Group 1998a, 1998b). Achieving these targets should be a priority in the management and prevention of CHD in UK Indian Asians (Department of Health 2000).

Insulin resistance is the key disturbance underlying increased CHD risk in UK Indian Asians (Mckeigue *et al.* 1991, 1993). However, a major limitation in the treatment of insulin resistance is the lack of solid evidence that improved insulin sensitivity is associated with a reduction in CHD mortality. Nevertheless, weight reduction, and increased physical activity are accepted measures to improve insulin sensitivity (Weinstock *et al.* 1998; Ross *et al.* 2000) and, in the future, novel insulin-sensitising agents, such as thiazolidinediones (Antonucci *et al.* 1997; Schoonjans & Auwerx 2000), may have important consequences in Indian Asians. Weight loss can be achieved merely by reducing the fat content of the diet without the need to restrict food intake voluntarily (Kendall *et al.* 1991). In UK Indian Asians, energy intake from fat is twice that of non-migrants (Mckeigue *et al.* 1985; Beegom *et al.* 1995). The most important practical measure is reducing the quantity of fat/oil used in preparation of foods. Most Indian Asians live in extended family units, and food is generally prepared at home. Targeted education of the 'shopper and cook' can be highly effective, and impact on other high-risk members of the family. Physical activity levels in Asians are low (Williams *et al.* 1994). Moderate activity including walking, swimming, cycling will have energy expenditures of about 100 kcal/h, and should be undertaken daily. It is important to maintain increased physical activity, otherwise the effects on insulin resistance are short-lived.

Implementation of measures

Prevention requires a multidisciplinary approach. Physicians should be motivated to translate available evidence from clinical studies into practice. Health economies, with large numbers of Indian Asians, should prioritise care, and ensure that resources are made available for clinicians to implement and audit accepted protocols. Coronary risk prevention teams should be equipped with suitable insights into methods of changing the varied Asian cultural subgroups. Most importantly, patients should have the information and education to make decisions, and be given 'ownership' of their risk factors as incentive, feedback and for regular reinforcement.

Conclusions and future directions

CHD in UK Indian Asians is preventable. Greatest benefit will be obtained from early and accurate diagnosis of CHD, and identification of those at increased risk. Aggressive correction of classic CHD risk factors, including cigarette smoking, dyslipidaemia and hypertension combined with intensive glycaemic control and control of obesity, should be the mainstay (Department of Health 2000). Reversal of insulin resistance is important – but not easily achieved or sustained. Until the 'magic bullet' is at hand systematic detection and correction of classic risk factors for CHD assumes even more importance in Indian Asians.

Future work is necessary to identify the precise environmental and genetic mechanisms underlying increased CHD risk in UK Indian Asians. Investigation of the heritability of metabolic disturbances within large, extended Indian Asian families may provide important insights into genetic factors determining CHD risk. The failure of the Framingham study risk predicts increased CHD risk in UK Indian Asians and also demonstrates the need for prospective population studies in Indian Asians to enable the development of strategies and risk prediction models that identify Indian Asians at increased CHD risk. Finally, novel treatment strategies are needed for subjects with insulin resistance, and controlled clinical trials are necessary to assess the effectiveness of treatment for insulin resistance, and other CHD risk factors, in this racial group.

References

Anand SS, Yusuf S, Vuksan V *et al.* (2000). Differences in risk factors, atherosclerosis, and cardiovascular disease between ethnic groups in Canada: the Study of Health Assessment and Risk in Ethnic groups (SHARE). *The Lancet* **356**, 279–284

Antonucci T, Whitcomb R, McLain R, Lockwood D, Norris RM (1997). Impaired glucose tolerance is normalized by treatment with the thiazolidinedione troglitazone. *Diabetes Care* **20**, 188–193

Assmann G, Schulte H, von Eckardstein A (1996). Hypertriglyceridemia and elevated lipoprotein(a) are risk factors for major coronary events in middle-aged men. *American Journal of Cardiology* **77**, 1179–1184

Balarajan R (1996). Ethnicity and variations in mortality from coronary heart disease. *Health Trends* **28**, 45–51

Beegom R, Beegom R, Niaz MA, Singh RB (1995). Diet, central obesity and prevalence of hypertension in the urban population of south India. *International Journal of Cardiology* **51**, 183–191

Bhatnagar D, Anand IS, Durrington PN *et al.* (1995). Coronary risk factors in people from the Indian subcontinent living in west London and their siblings in India. *The Lancet* **345**, 405–409

Bhopal R, Unwin N, White M *et al.* (1999). Heterogeneity of coronary heart disease risk factors in Indian, Pakistani, Bangladeshi, and European origin populations: cross sectional study. *British Medical Journal* **319**, 215–220

Boerwinkle E, Leffert CC, Lin J, Lackner C, Chiesa G, Hobbs HH (1992). Apolipoprotein(a) gene accounts for greater than 90 per cent of the variation in plasma lipoprotein(a) concentrations. *Journal of Clinical Investigations* **90**, 52–60

British Cardic Society *et al.* (1998). Joint British recommendations on prevention of coronary heart disease in clinical practice. *Heart* **80**, S1–29

Chambers JC & Kooner JS (2000). C-reactive protein and coronary heart disease risk in UK Indian Asians, compared to European whites. *Heart* **83**, 50

Chambers JC, Obeid OA, Refsum H *et al.* (2000a). Plasma homocysteine concentrations and risk of coronary heart disease in UK Indian Asian and European men. *The Lancet* **355**, 523–527

Chambers JC, Wrigley J, Kooner JS (2000b). Evaluation of the Joint British Societies coronary heart disease risk calculator in UK Indian Asians. *Heart* **43**

Chambers JC, Ireland H, Thompson E *et al.* (2001). The methylenetetrahydrofolate reductase 677 C→T mutation, and coronary heart disease risk in UK Indian Asians. *Arteriosclerosis Thrombosis and Vascular Biology* in press

Department of Health (2000). *National Service Framework for Coronary Heart Disease.* London: Stationery Office

Downs JR, Clearfield M, Weis S *et al.* (1998). Primary prevention of acute coronary events with lovastatin in men and women with average cholesterol levels: results of AFCAPS/TexCAPS. Air Force/Texas Coronary Atherosclerosis Prevention Study. *Journal of the American Medical Association* **279**, 1615–1622

Hansson L, Zanchetti A, Carruthers SG *et al.* (1998). Effects of intensive blood-pressure lowering and low-dose aspirin in patients with hypertension: principal results of the Hypertension Optimal Treatment (HOT) randomised trial. HOT Study Group. *The Lancet* **351**, 1755–1762

Harper CR & Jacobson TA (1999). New perspectives on the management of low levels of high-density lipoprotein cholesterol. *Archives of Internal Medicine* **159**, 1049–1057

Haverkate F, Thompson SG, Pyke SD, Gallimore JR, Pepys MB (1997). Production of C-reactive protein and risk of coronary events in stable and unstable angina. European Concerted Action on Thrombosis and Disabilities Angina Pectoris Study Group. *The Lancet* **349**, 462–426

Kaplan NM (1992). Systolic hypertension in the elderly program (SHEP) and Swedish trial in old patients with hypertension (STOP). The promises and the potential problems. *American Journal of Hypertension* **5**, 331–334

Kendall A, Levitsky DA, Strupp BJ, Lissner L (1991). Weight loss on a low-fat diet: consequence of the imprecision of the control of food intake in humans. *American Journal of Clinical Nutrition* **53**, 1124–1129

Kooner JS, Baliga RR, Wilding J *et al.* (1998). Abdominal obesity, impaired nonesterified fatty acid suppression, and insulin-mediated glucose disposal are early metabolic abnormalities in families with premature myocardial infarction. *Arteriosclerosis Thrombosis and Vascular Biology* **18**, 1021–1026

Leaverton PE, Sorlie PD, Kleinman JC *et al.* (1987). Representativeness of the Framingham risk model for coronary heart disease mortality: a comparison with a national cohort study. *Journal of Chronic Diseases* **40**, 775–784

Mather HM & Keen H (1985). The Southall Diabetes Survey: prevalence of known diabetes in Asians and Europeans. *British Medical Journal* **291**, 1081–1084

Mather HM, Chaturvedi N, Fuller JH (1998). Mortality and morbidity from diabetes in South Asians and Europeans: 11-year follow-up of the Southall Diabetes Survey, London, UK. *Diabetic Medicine* **15**, 53–59

McKeigue PM, Ferrie JE, Pierpoint T, Marmot MG (1993). Association of early-onset coronary heart disease in South Asian men with glucose intolerance and hyperinsulinemia. *Circulation* **87**, 152–161

McKeigue PM, Marmot MG, Adelstein AM *et al.* (1985). Diet and risk factors for coronary heart disease in Asians in northwest London. *The Lancet* **ii**, 1086–1090

McKeigue PM, Shah B, Marmot MG (1991). Relation of central obesity and insulin resistance with high diabetes prevalence and cardiovascular risk in South Asians. *The Lancet* **337**, 382–386

Pais P, Pogue J, Gerstein H *et al.* (1996). Risk factors for acute myocardial infarction in Indians: a case- control study. *The Lancet* **348**, 358–363

Ridker PM, Hennekens CH, Buring JE, Rifai N (2000). C-reactive protein and other markers of inflammation in the prediction of cardiovascular disease in women. *New England Journal of Medicine* **342**, 836–843

Ross R (1999). Atherosclerosis-an inflammatory disease. *New England Journal of Medicine* **340**, 115–126

Ross R, Dagnone D, Jones PJ *et al.* (2000). Reduction in obesity and related comorbid conditions after diet-induced weight loss or exercise-induced weight loss in men. A randomized, controlled trial. *Annals of Internal Medicine* **133**, 92–103

Rubins HB, Robins SJ, Collins D *et al.* (1999). Gemfibrozil for the secondary prevention of coronary heart disease in men with low levels of high-density lipoprotein cholesterol. Veterans Affairs High-Density Lipoprotein Cholesterol Intervention Trial Study Group. *New England Journal of Medicine* **341**, 410–418

Sacks FM, Pfeffer MA, Moye LA *et al.* (1996). The effect of pravastatin on coronary events after myocardial infarction in patients with average cholesterol levels. Cholesterol and Recurrent Events Trial investigators. *New England Journal of Medicine* **335**, 1001–1009

Schoonjans K & Auwerx J (2000). Thiazolidinediones: an update. *The Lancet* **355**, 1008–1010

The Long-term Intervention with Pravastatin in Ischaemic Disease (LIPID) Study Group (1998). Prevention of cardiovascular events and death with pravastatin in patients with coronary heart disease and a broad range of initial cholesterol levels. *New England Journal of Medicine* **339**, 1349–1357

UK Prospective Diabetes Study (UKPDS) Group (1998a). Effect of intensive blood-glucose control with metformin on complications in overweight patients with type 2 diabetes (UKPDS 34). *The Lancet* **352**, 854–865

UK Prospective Diabetes Study (UKPDS) Group (1998b). Intensive blood-glucose control with sulphonylureas or insulin compared with conventional treatment and risk of complications in patients with type 2 diabetes (UKPDS 33). *The Lancet* **352**, 837–853

van den Hoogen PC, Feskens EJ, Nagelkerke NJ, Menotti A, Nissinen A, Kromhout D (2000). The relation between blood pressure and mortality due to coronary heart disease among men in different parts of the world. Seven Countries Study Research Group. *New England Journal of Medicine* **342**, 1–8

Weinstock RS, Dai H, Wadden TA (1998). Diet and exercise in the treatment of obesity: effects of 3 interventions on insulin resistance. *Archives of Internal Medicine* **158**, 2477–2483

Wilkinson P, Sayer J, Laji K *et al.* (1996). Comparison of case fatality in south Asian and white patients after acute myocardial infarction: observational study. *British Medical Journal* **312**, 1330–1333

Williams R, Bhopal R, Hunt K (1994). Coronary risk in a British Punjabi population: comparative profile of non-biochemical factors. *International Journal of Epidemiology* **23**, 28–37

Wood D, De Backer G, Faergeman O, Graham I, Mancia G, Pyorala K (1998). Prevention of coronary heart disease in clinical practice: recommendations of the Second Joint Task Force of European and other Societies on Coronary Prevention. *Atherosclerosis* **140**, 199–270

Yudkin JS, Stehouwer CD, Emeis JJ, Coppack SW (1999). C-reactive protein in healthy subjects: associations with obesity, insulin resistance, and endothelial dysfunction: a potential role for cytokines originating from adipose tissue? *Arterioscleosis Thrombosis and Vascular Biology* **19**, 972–978

Chapter 9

Ensuring patient benefit from effective services: the issues of access and equity

Hugh JN Bethell

Introduction

The general practitioner is the key to both access and equity in the provision of secondary prevention of coronary disease. Nearly all secondary prevention is carried out in primary care. The paradox is that general practitioners are rarely consulted about secondary prevention. Take, for example, the latest set of guidelines produced by the British Cardiac Society, the British Hypertension Society, the British Hyperlipidaemia Association and the British Diabetic Association (Wood *et al.* 1998), guidelines that are to be used almost exclusively in general practice. Not a single general practitioner is included in the long list of contributors.

If the medical establishment cannot see the importance of primary care as the vehicle for secondary prevention of coronary disease it is hardly surprising that successive governments have also failed to grasp the point.

In 1993, the government replaced Kenneth Clark's Health Promotion Clinic scheme for general practice with the 'Banding' system of health promotion. General practitioners were paid for providing services or collecting information under three bands with increasing payment for each extra band covered. Hidden in Band 2, among such dubious activities as the recording of patients' height and weight and exercise habit, was the requirement to provide structured care for patients with coronary disease, hypertension and cerebrovascular disease. The care of asthma and diabetes mellitus was not included in the Banding system but each was given its own 'Chronic disease management' funding. It is ironic that the chronic disease that kills more people than any other in the UK was not thought important enough to warrant separate financing.

The National Service Framework (NSF) for Coronary Heart Disease, Standard 3 (Department of Health 2000) has at last recognised the importance of general practice as the overseer of secondary prevention.

The bones of the problem are clear:

1. Secondary prevention of coronary disease is effective.
2. Secondary prevention is not currently being provided properly in general practice.
3. Ways of improving the situation must be found.

Secondary prevention is effective

The following measures have been shown to improve the prognosis of patients with CHD:

- Stopping smoking: those patients who stop smoking cigarettes after a myocardial infarction have half the risk of future infarction of those who continue (Aberg *et al.* 1983). The advice of general practitioners is one of the most cost-effective ways of getting patients to quit the habit (Chapman 1993).
- Low-dose aspirin: long-term low-dose aspirin reduces future coronary events in patients with CHD by about 20 per cent (Antiplatelets Triallists' Collaboration 1994).
- β Blockade: after myocardial infarction β blockade also reduces the incidence of future events by about 20 per cent (Beta-blocker Heart Attack Trial Research Group 1982).
- Blood cholesterol reduction: the use of statins to treat mildly raised blood cholesterol levels in patients with CHD who are already on an optimal diet reduces infarction by 46 per cent and mortality by 30 per cent (Scandinavian Simvastatin Survival Study 1994).
- Treatment of hypertension: the protection against coronary disease produced by hypotensive medication, although less than against stroke, is still substantial (Collins *et al.* 1990).
- Angiotensin-converting enzyme (ACE) inhibition in coronary patients with poor left ventricular function (Yusuf *et al.* 1992; AIRE Study Investigators 1993).
- Exercise-based cardiac rehabilitation: meta-analyses of the randomised controlled trials of cardiac rehabilitation have shown a reduction in mortality in treated groups of between 20 and 25 per cent (Oldridge *et al.* 1988; O'Connor *et al.* 1989).

Secondary prevention, targeting as it does those at high risk, is very cost-effective (Oldridge *et al.* 1993). An analysis of the factors behind the fall in coronary mortality in the USA has indicated that 75 per cent of the reduction is due to treatment and preventive measures for coronary patients and only 25 per cent is due to primary prevention activities (Hunink *et al.* 1997).

Secondary prevention is not currently being adequately provided in general practice

The ASPIRE study (Bowker *et al.* 1996) showed that secondary prevention was not being properly applied in hospital practice even by cardiologists (Bethell 1997). The position in general practice is likely to be substantially worse. There are several measures that are known to improve prognosis in coronary disease and that have been shown as not being implemented in general practice:

1. A large minority of coronary patients do not take prophylactic aspirin (McCallum *et al.* 1997).
2. β Blockade is greatly underused after myocardial infarction (Eccles & Bradshaw 1991).
3. The control of blood cholesterol in post-infarct patients has been shown to be inadequate, with the implication that many lives could be saved if this were corrected (Feder *et al.* 1999).
4. Only between one-half and one-third of hypertensive patients have adequate treatment for their disease (Mancia *et al.* 1997).
5. ACE inhibitors are underused in patients who should benefit from their prescription. One study found that 37 per cent of a group of patients who suffered heart failure after myocardial infarction were not given these drugs (Bradley *et al.* 1997).
6. Less than 20 per cent of patients following myocardial infarction are enrolled in exercise-based cardiac rehabilitation programmes (Horgan *et al.* 1992; Campbell *et al.* 1996). General practitioners, as purchasers and commissioners of care, are in a good position to lobby for increased provision of this underfunded treatment.

Some of these deficiencies are addressed by the National Service Framework for Coronary Heart Disease (Department of Health 2000) which expects 90 per cent of coronary patients to take aspirin, 80 per cent β blockers and 80 per cent statins. The document also supports the much wider and more complete provision of cardiac rehabilitation (Standard 12) and intends that more than 85 per cent of patients discharged from hospital following acute myocardial infarction or coronary revascularisation should be offered cardiac rehabilitation.

It is important to recognise that some interventions are likely to fail and, while not ignoring them, not expect healthcare professionals to spend too much time or resources on them. They are discussed below.

1. Cigarette smoking: having a heart attack is a powerful aid to giving up smoking – but those who fail to stop at the time of the attack are very unlikely to succeed later. I cannot remember one exception to this.
2. Healthy eating: weight loss is the exception for the recovering patient. Those who have given up smoking will almost certainly gain weight. Fat patients tend to get fatter and thin patients may get thinner after a heart attack. Diet alone seldom leads to a reduction in blood cholesterol – probably because patients find it too difficult to change their eating habits. One memorable study – by Nikolaus *et al.* (1991) – found that not only did coronary patients fail to adhere to low-fat diets but also they lied to the investigators about what they were eating. Two randomised controlled trials of cholesterol-lowering diets in coronary patients have shown a reduction in the treated group – the St Thomas'

Atherosclerosis Regression Study (Watts *et al.* 1992) and the Lyon Diet Heart Study (Lorgeril *et al.* 1994). In both cases the patients not only received enormous amounts of dietitian time but also were given some of the ingredients of their recommended diet. Only Ornish *et al.* (1990) inspired his congregation with the necessary evangelical fervour to reduce their blood cholesterols by their own efforts.

3. Independent exercise: exercise levels are definitely increased by cardiac rehabilitation programmes but there is a high default rate after the end of the supervised course. Individual exercise prescription is likely to fail. The Newcastle exercise project (Harland *et al.* 1999) used three strategies to increase exercising among 40- to 64-year-old adults. Even paying the patient to use leisure facilities failed to increase the level of exercise at one year.

Although part of the deficiency lies in failure of hospital treatment, the long-term care of coronary patients is the province of the general practitioner. Patients with coronary artery disease are suffering from a chronic progressive condition and they should be followed up at regular intervals to check on symptoms, lifestyle, risk factors and treatment (Bethell 1996). This is hardly ever done in hospital outpatients.

Improving the situation

Start right

Most of the coronary patients whose chronic management falls to the GP have been through the hospital system. GPs, on the whole, continue the treatment initiated by the hospital and it is essential that patients be discharged from secondary care on optimal medication. The importance of failures at this crucial stage is not always recognised.

The POST Study (Feder *et al.* 1999) looked at the management of 328 patients from Hackney in east London who had been admitted to hospital with myocardial infarction or unstable angina. The 59 practices with whom they were registered were randomised to intervention or control groups. The intervention consisted of postal prompts to both GP and patient. The outcomes included the proportion of patients on β blockers at six months and the proportion on cholesterol lowerers at one year. For these outcomes there were no differences between the groups with combined group prescribing of β blockers at only 33 per cent and of cholesterol lowerers of only 24 per cent. The possibility that the patients had not been discharged on appropriate medication was not even considered by the authors, most of whom were GPs. One reason for the failure of hospitals is the fact that acute infarct patients are admitted to hospital under the care of the on-duty physician whose main interest is likely to be lung disease, endocrinology, kidney disease, gastroenterology or just possibly cardiology.

In January 1999, the Coronary Prevention Group Secondary Prevention and Rehabilitation Committee carried out a questionnaire survey of all the 325 coronary care units (CCUs) in the UK (Bethell *et al.* 1999), asking under whose care acute infarct patients were admitted and whether the patients had access to a cardiological opinion. There was a 75 per cent response.

In 40 per cent, infarct patients were admitted under the care of a cardiologist or physician with an interest in cardiology. In the remaining 60 per cent, patients were admitted under the care of the duty general physician. Most had access to a cardiologist's opinion but this was not available in 6 per cent. Follow-up was provided by a cardiac clinic in 21 per cent and a specific cardiac rehabilitation clinic in 17 per cent, but the remainder were seen in the general medical out-patient clinic. The Nottingham study of the progress of 900 infarct patients, however, found that 18 per cent did not even receive a follow-up appointment (Melville *et al.* 1999).

The first necessity for the effective long-term management of coronary patients is that they be seen by a cardiologist or physician with an interest in cardiology during their recovery from the acute event, so that their future drug treatment can be optimised and further investigations including angiography can be planned. It is heartening that the NSF document recommends that all infarct patients should receive the opinion of a cardiologist.

Ensure attendance at a cardiac rehabilitation clinic – if it exists

The meta-analyses of randomised controlled trials of cardiac rehabilitation have all agreed that multidisciplinary rehabilitation reduces mortality by about 20 per cent over the three years following acute infarction. Currently there are about 280 cardiac rehabilitation centres in the UK covering about 80 per cent of the population. Unfortunately the number of patients treated in each falls far short of the number who might benefit. The recent British Association for Cardiac Rehabilitation survey of units in the UK came to the conclusion that about 20 per cent of infarct patients are enrolled and about 45 per cent of coronary artery bypass graft patients but only 8 per cent of percutaneous transluminal coronary angioplasty patients (Bethell *et al.* 2001). There is plenty of room for improvement which will only come with better funding of existing programmes.

Organise nurse-run follow-up clinics in general practice

Patients who have recovered from an acute coronary event are followed up in general practice. Good systems are needed to ensure that all such patients receive the benefits of evidence-based secondary prevention alluded to earlier.

On the whole doctors are not particularly good at following protocols. A successful protocol needs to be clearly written as a computer template and followed by a nurse.

Trials of secondary prevention have shown improvements in patient statements about their health and their health-improving habits. Cupples and McKnight (1994) performed a randomised controlled trial of health education in 688 patients with angina. They found that, after two years, the treated group reported taking more exercise, eating a healthier diet and suffering less angina than the controls. However, there were no differences in smoking habit, blood pressure, blood cholesterol or body mass index (BMI). The improvements had largely evaporated after five years (Cupples & McKnight 1999). Campbell *et al.* (1998) randomised 1,173 patients with CHD into a clinic system run by nurses and after one year found improvements in various domains of the SF-36 scale and lessening of angina, but not of anxiety or depression. They did, however, find a reduced hospital admission rate in the treated group. More recently the SHIP study (Jolly *et al.* 1999) randomised practices in Southampton into intervention and control groups – the intervention practices to receive visits from a liaison cardiac nurse with encouragement to provide structured follow-up for their patients with new angina or recent myocardial infarct. At one year there were no differences between the groups for lipid levels, blood pressure, fitness or smoking habit. The POST study (Feder *et al.* 1999) used postal prompts to both patients and their GPs (who had been sent reminders of effective interventions and the existence of local guidelines for coronary disease), randomised by practice. It failed to show any improvement in the initially low level of prescribing of β blockers or lipid lowerers.

The SHIP investigators concluded: 'Ischaemic heart disease is a chronic condition which requires the same systematic approach to secondary prevention applied in other chronic conditions such as diabetes mellitus.'

Written guidelines are helpful but the Cochrane Systematic review found that they do little to change health professionals' behaviour (Freemantle *et al.* 1977). However, computer templates or 'computer-based clinical reminder systems' have been shown to improve patient care (Shea *et al.* 1996; Marriott 1999).

The great majority of general practitioners have computers on their desks and a handful of companies provide the software for their use. This usually includes templates for the management of a variety of situations such as initial health checks, contraception protocols, chronic disease management strategies, etc. The templates available for the management of coronary disease are of variable and often inferior quality.

A template for secondary prevention (Figure 9.1)

The Secondary Prevention and Rehabilitation Advisory Committee of the Coronary Prevention Group has devised a template which the author believes is simple and short enough to be usable in consultation by either the practice nurse or the GP, and comprehensive enough to cover the important points for secondary prevention.

ISCHAEMIC HEART DISEASE

DATABASE

* EVENT	*n*	Date
	Angina pectoris	from:
	Myocardial infarct	1:
		2:
		3:
	PTCA	1:
		2:
		3:
	CABG	1:
		2:

CHANGEABLE RISK FACTORS AT ONSET

* Cigarette smoking	Current smoker	
	Ex-smoker	
	Never smoked	
* Height:		....
* Weight		....
BMI	....	
* Blood pressure	Syst	....
	Diast	....
* Total cholesterol		....
LDL		....
HDL		....
Ratio		....
Fasting trigylceride		....
* Sugar		....
*TSH		....
*Urine		....

Figure 9.1 The template

FOLLOW-UP DATA

SYMPTOMS

* Cigarette smoking	Current smoker	
	Ex-smoker	
	Never smoked	
* Angina	Nil	
	With severe exertion	
	With moderate exertion	
	With light effort	
	At rest/Nocturnal	
* Breathlessness	Nil	(NYHA GD I)
	With moderate exercise	(NYHA GD II)
	With light exertion	(NYHA GD III)
	At rest	(NYHA GD IV)
	Hours/week	
Exercise habit	Adequate	
	Inadequate	
	(if inadequate, PIL triggered)	

Signs

* Weight		....
BMI	....	
* Blood pressure	syst	....
	diast	....

Investigations

* Cholesterol	....
LDL	....
HDL	....
Ratio	....
Triglyceride	....
* Urine	....

Treatment

* Asprin	Y/N	If N – contraindicated text ....
* Beta blocker	Y/N	If N – contraindicated text ....
* Lipid lowerer	Y/N	If N – contraindicated text ....
* ACE inhibitor	Y/N	If N – not indicated contraindicated

Does the patient need referral back to the GP Y/N

Follow-up 1 year

* Starred items will continue to flash until completed.

Figure 9.1 The template (continued)

The initial database includes a list of acute coronary events which may be added to from time to time and a list of changeable risk factors at the time of first diagnosis.

The follow-up chart includes symptoms, signs, investigations and treatment – items that should be responded to annually will flash until completed.

Hospital IT systems record coronary patient data. The British Heart Foundation is developing stand-alone computer support software for use by cardiac rehabilitation co-ordinators. It is essential that all these systems are designed to talk to each other so that information moves smoothly from the hospital through the rehabilitation programme to the GP.

Conclusion

The author believes that the most effective way of implementing coronary secondary prevention in general practice will be through nurse-run clinics backed up by evidence-based computer templates. The chronic disease management of asthma has set an example of the effectiveness of this approach.

Since 1993, the regular surveillance of asthma patients has been rewarded with a 'chronic disease management' payment. The use of specially trained asthma nurses for this purpose has been widespread. There has been a significant improvement in the treatment of asthma with an increase in use of prophylactic inhaled steroids and a fall in acute admissions. Despite an increase in the prevalence of asthma, mortality from asthma in the UK is declining (Campbell *et al.* 1997). This improvement is certainly linked with an improvement in care provided by GPs.

New money should be made available for the employment of trained cardiac nurses to run similar chronic disease management clinics for the management of coronary disease, thus ensuring both ready access and equity of access.

References

Aberg A, Berestrand R, Johansson S *et al.* (1983). Cessation of smoking after myocardial infarction: effects on mortality after 10 years. *British Heart Journal* **49**, 416–422

Acute Infarction Ramipril Efficacy (AIRE) Study Investigators (1993). Effect of ramipril on mortality and morbidity of survivors of acute MI with evidence of heart failure. *The Lancet* **342**, 821–828

Antiplatelet Trialists' Collaboration (1994). Collaborative overviews of randomised controlled trials of antiplatelet therapy. I: Prevention of death, myocardial infarction and stroke by prolonged antiplatelet therapy in various categories of patients. *British Medical Journal* **308**, 81–106

Beta-blocker Heart Attack Trial Research Group (1982). A randomised trial of propranolol in patients with acute myocardial infarction. *Journal of the American Medical Association* **247**, 1707

Bethell HJN (1996). Going home. The first few weeks after a heart attack. *British Medical Journal* **312**, 1372

Bethell HJN (1997). Coronary patients need cardiologists. *Heart* **77**, 389

Bethell H, Graham R, Wallwork M (1999). The POST Study: a failure of hospitals not GPs. www.bmj.com/cgl/eletters/318/7197/1522

Bethell HJN, Turner SC, Evans JA, Rose L (2001). Cardiac rehabilitation in the United Kingdom. How complete is the provision? *Journal of Cardiopulmonary Rehabilitation* **21**, 111–115

Bowker T, Clayton TC, Ingham J *et al.* (1996). A British Cardiac Society survey of the potential for secondary prevention of coronary disease: ASPIRE (Action on Secondary Prevention through Intervention to Reduce Events). *Heart* **75**, 334–342

Bradley F, Morgan S, Smith H, Mant D (1997). Preventive care for patients following myocardial infarction. *Family Practice* **14**, 220–226

Campbell MJ, Cogman GR, Holgate ST, Johnston SL (1997). Age specific trends in asthma mortality in England and Wales, 1983-95: results of an observational study. *British Medical Journal* **314**, 1439–1441

Campbell NC, Grimshaw JM, Ritchie LD, Rawles JM (1996). Outpatient cardiac rehabilitation: are the potential benefits being realised? *Journal of the Royal College of Physicians* **30**, 514–519

Campbell NC, Thain J, Deans HG *et al.* (1998). Secondary prevention clinics for coronary heart disease: randomised trial of effect on health. *British Medical Journal* **316**, 1434–1437

Chapman S (1993). The role of doctors in promoting smoking cessation. *British Medical Journal* **307**, 518

Collins R, Peto C, MacMahon S *et al.* (1990). Blood, pressure, stroke and coronary heart disease. Part 2: Short term reductions in blood pressure: overview of randomised trials in their epidemiological context. *The Lancet* **335**, 827–838

Cupples ME & McKnight A (1994). A randomised controlled trial of health promotion in general practice for patients at high cardiovascular risk. *British Medical Journal* **309**, 993–996

Cupples ME & McKnight A (1999). Five year follow up of patients as high cardiovascular risk who took part in randomised controlled of health promotion. *British Medical Journal* **319**, 687–688

Department of Health (2000). *National Service Frameworks. Coronary Heart Disease.* London: HMSO

Eccles M & Bradshaw C (1991). Use of secondary prophylaxis after myocardial infarction in the North of England. *British Medical Journal* **302**, 91–92

Feder G, Griffiths C, Eldridge S, Spence M (1999). Effect of postal prompts to patients and general practitioners on the quality of primary care after a coronary event (POST): randomised controlled trial. *British Medical Journal* **318**, 1522–1526

Freemantle N, Harvey EL, Grimshaw JM *et al.* (1997). The effectiveness of printed educational materials in changing the behaviour of healthcare professionals. The Cochrane Database of Systematic Reviews

Harland J, White M, Drinkwater C *et al.* (1999). The Newcastle exercise project: a randomised controlled trial of methods to promote physical activity in primary care. *British Medical Journal* **319**, 828–832

Horgan J, Bethell H, Carson P *et al.* (1992). British Cardiac Society working party report on cardiac rehabilitation. *British Heart Journal* **67**, 412–418

Hunink MGM, Goldman L, Tosteson ANA *et al.* (1997). The recent decline in mortality from coronary heart disease, 1980–1990. The effect of secular trends in risk factors and treatment. *Journal of the American Medical Association* **277**, 535–542

Jolly K, Bradley F, Sharp S *et al.* (1999). Randomised controlled trial of follow up care in general practice of patients with myocardial infarction and angina: final results of the Southampton heart integrated care project (SHIP). *British Medical Journal* **318**, 706–711

Lorgeril M, Renaud S, Mamell N *et al.* (1994). Meditarrenean aplha-lilonelic acid-rich diet in secondary prevention of coronary heart disease. *The Lancet* **343**, 1454–1459

Mancia G, Sega R, Milesi C *et al.* (1997). Blood-pressure in the hypertensive population. *The Lancet* **i**, 454–457

Marriott R (1999). Opportunistic screening for the secondary prevention of coronary artery disease (Abst). *Journal of Integrated Care* **3**, 46

McCallum AK, Whincup PH, Morris RW *et al.* (1997). Aspirin use in middle-aged men with cardiovascular disease: are opportunities being missed? *British Journal of General Practice* **47**, 417–421

Melville M, Brown N Gray D, Young T, Hampton J (1999). Outcome and use of health services four years after admission for acute myocardial infarction: case record follow up study. *British Medical Journal* **319**, 231–232

Nikolaus T, Schlierf G, Vogel G, Schuler G, Wagner I (1991). Treatment of coronary heart disease with diet and exercise – problems of compliance. *Annals of Nutrition and Metabolism* **35**, 1–7

O'Connor G, Buring J, Yusuf S *et al.* (1989). An overview of randomised trials of rehabilitation with exercise after myocardial infarction. *Circulation* **80**, 234–244

Oldridge N, Guyatt G, Fischer M, Rimm A (1988). Cardiac rehabilitation after myocardial infarction. Combined experience of randomised clinical trials. *Journal of the American Medical Association* **260**, 945–950

Oldridge N, Furlong W, Feeny D *et al.* (1993). Economic evaluation cardiac rehabilitation soon after acute myocardial infarction. *American Journal of Cardiology* **72**, 154–161

Ornish D, Brown SE, Scherwitz LW *et al.* (1990). Can lifestyle changes reverse coronary heart disease? The Lifestyle Heart Trial. *The Lancet* **336**, 129–133

Scandinavian Simvastatin Survival Study Group (1994). Randomised trial of cholesterol lowering in 4,444 patients with coronary artery disease. *The Lancet* **344**, 1393–1399

Shea S, DuMouchel W, Bahamonde L (1996). A meta-analysis of 16 randomised controlled trials to evaluate computer-based clinical reminder systems for preventive care in the ambulatory setting. *Journal of the American Medical Information Association* **3**, 399–409

Watts GF, Lewis B, Brunt JNH *et al.* (1992). Effects on coronary artery disease of lipid lowering diet, or diet plus cholestyramine, in the St Thomas' atherosclerosis Regression Study (STARS). *The Lancet* **339**, 563–569

Wood D, Durrington P, Poulter *et al.* (1998). Joint British recommendations on prevention of coronary heart disease in clinical practice. *Heart* **80**, Suppl 2

Yusuf S, Pepone C, Garces C *et al.* (1992). Effect of enalapril on myocardial infarction and unstable angina in patients with low ejection fraction. *The Lancet* **340**, 1173–1178

Index